Sports Nutrition

The Base Manual For Obtaining Maximum Performance

Table of Contents

Introduction

Congratulations on downloading your personal copy of *Sports Nutrition: The Base Manual For Obtaining Maximum Performance*. Thank you for doing so.

The following chapters will discuss how the proper diet will improve performance in exercise, and will give you more energy both on and off the field. Certain nutrition regimens can be used to naturally enhance performance for endurance sports like running and biking. Moreover, weight bearing sports like professional weight lifting and contact sports like football also improve proficiency.

You will discover how important a well balanced diet is to overall well being and physical performance.

The following chapters will explore variation diets specifically for your exercise of choice, and general guidelines for improved nutrition for everyone.

There are plenty of books on this subject on the market, thanks again for choosing this one! Every effort was made to ensure it is full of as much useful information as possible. Please enjoy!

Congratulations on downloading your personal copy of the *Sports Nutrition: The base manual for obtaining maximum performance*. Thank you for doing so.

Chapter 1: Check your health

Whether starting a brand new exercise routine or you want to improve your strength or endurance with your current plan or sport, good nutrition is where it starts. Two main types of exercise will be discussed here; endurance training and weight training.

In general, endurance training is considered as any sort of aerobic exercise, like running, jogging, dancing or swimming. Any exercise that increases the heart rate is aerobic exercise, and when done for long periods of time, takes a great deal of endurance from the heart, lungs and limbs.

Weight training is non-aerobic exercise, although the heart rate does increase during these exercises as well. Generally, it takes less oxygen from the lungs to work the muscles when using free weights and working on specific muscle groups, rather than with endurance training.

Whatever exercise you participate in, it is a good idea to check in regularly with your doctor or health care provider to make sure your body is fit for activity. Your doctor will check for signs that your heart or lungs are strained and unfit for exercise. Before beginning a regimen, have your doctor monitor your heart rate, and breathing patterns, do blood tests to check your blood sugar, cholesterol and other panels to pinpoint any underlying problems. Most likely, if you have no signs or symptoms of a problem, the doctor won't find anything either, but better safe than sorry. Overdoing it can easily overwhelm your system, causing you to faint or have other unwanted symptoms.

The good news is, doing any sort of exercise routine will improve all of those lab values, so getting a baseline for your health status before you begin will be a good comparison point further on in your exercise plan. Seeing as most people exercise for the benefit of their health, this is a useful tool.

Chapter 2: Developing an exercise regimen

When planning to start something new or improve upon your current routine, make sure to start small as to not overwhelm your body. For example, if you currently are mainly sedentary, working a desk job with little activity during the day, expecting to run five miles, or even a mile, is quite a lofty goal. Instead, plan to begin your exercise routine in a stepwise fashion, making small goals that will eventually lead to your ultimate goal. In this case, making your initial goal to walk a mile five days a week would be a more reasonable start. After awhile, your stamina will build up, and you will begin jogging, then running, then for longer distances, but it all starts with modest increases to preserve the integrity of your body.

For those who already have a steady exercise program down, or participate in regular sports are likely ready to improve their performance, and that begins with small goals as well. Studies have shown that muscles memorize certain movements and exercises, and begin to do them with less energy as they are done more and more. This is a good and a bad thing, depending on your goal. If you are a professional athlete, say, a soccer player, muscle memory will work well in your favor. However, if you are on a weight loss program and your muscles begin to get comfortable with your routine, they will use less energy, and you will not be able to continue losing weight like you were.

Either way, switching up your workout routine, changing the order of exercise or trying something new will keep your muscles on their toes and your workout, and your endurance, will begin to improve. As you get comfortable, increase the weight, increase the repetitions, then change things up again. An exercise routine is nothing if it cannot be variable, changing at any given time.

No matter what your activity of choice is, adding something to your routine is good but make a plan for yourself. Use the following chapters to develop a well rounded nutrition plan for yourself that fits in line with your exercise plan. Use these tips and tools to plan an ideal menu for your activity level. In general, a normal healthy person requires 25-30 calories per kilogram of weight, plus the estimated amount that will be used for energy. For example, a 200 pound person will require 2250-2700 calories, plus what could be lost during exercise to maintain their current weight. The number of calories burned during exercise is highly variable, based on weight and fitness level.

For help determining an appropriate calorie level and macronutrient ratio, consult with a registered dietitian or nutritionist for individualized help. Adding exercise will increase the overall energy needs of the body, and it is important to match your eating plan with your activity level. Again, please consult with a health care professional to determine if adding exercise to your current lifestyle is safe and appropriate for you.

Chapter 3: Basic nutrition for athletes of all shapes and forms

Before getting into the minute details of endurance or weight training, it is important to understand the basis of a well rounded, nutritious diet in general. Think of your body as a machine. In order to run properly, a machine needs, oils and gases to fuel it, and the same is true with your body. The body's fuel is food, and just like premium versus regular gas, not all food is created equal.

Let's start simply, with the look of your plate. Every person, athlete or not should base their plate around vegetables. Half of the plate should consist of non-starchy veggies like lettuce, tomato, cucumber, zucchini and many more. The key word here is non-starchy, which would not include potatoes, corn or winter squashes, as these vegetables would be considered a carbohydrate.

The other half of the plate should be split between your carbohydrate, like the potato, and a lean protein like chicken breast or steak. The exact portion sizes will vary depending on your individual calorie needs, but by simply portioning your foods in this ratio will be a good start. Consult with a health care professional to determine what your specific calorie needs are.

When it comes to protein, finding good quality, lean cut of meat, or using non-animal sources like beans and quinoa for protein, is essential. Avoid fatty proteins like bacon, dark meat poultry, and high fat ground beef, as they contain higher amounts of saturated fat than leaner cuts, and can add unneeded calories, and can raise your blood cholesterol. The source of meat is also important. Grass fed organic meats are of best quality because the meat is raised without antibiotics or other chemicals that are passed into the meat. Also, when animals are fed their natural diet, like grass for cows, the meat is of better quality, higher in anti-inflammatory Omega 3 fatty acids.

Meat from grain-fed animals is higher in pro-inflammatory Omega 6 fatty acids, which can be detrimental to the body in excessive amounts. These Omega 6 fatty acids are also found in grain products in abundance, so they are not necessary in your meat as well.

Chapter 4: How does food work in the body?

With nutrition, it is important to understand how different types of foods act within the body. There are three main macronutrients; protein, carbohydrates and fat. Each can be used for fuel in the body, but use different mechanisms to do so.

Carbohydrates are the body's preferred source of fuel. The simple sugars that make up carbohydrates are quickly and easily broken down into energy, which can be used right away. In fact, carbohydrates serve no other purpose in the body except for fuel. Any excess carbs that cannot be used for energy at that time will be stored as fat in the body for use later.

This is the reason that low carbohydrate diets are often recommended for weight loss. Giving the body only what it needs stops the production of fat, and forces the body to use stores that it has built up, rather than continually providing excess through the diet. Heavy carbs like potatoes and pasta should be limited, while lower carb fruits should be chosen in their place. Fruits also provide fiber, which cannot be broken down and used for energy, but helps keep the digestive tract moving.

Protein molecules are the building blocks of muscle. Proteins from the body are broken down into amino acids, which help build and repair muscles. Protein from animals like chicken and cows, as well as plant proteins like beans are both necessary for muscle growth, but animal proteins provide more of the essential amino acids needed for healthy muscles.

Dietary fat is also a necessary nutrient, and per gram, provides the most energy of the three macronutrients. In the past, it was thought that dietary fat was solely responsible for increasing fat stores in the body. We now know that is untrue, as excess carbohydrates are more a culprit for fat storage than dietary fats. In the body, fats are necessary to aid in the digestion of fat soluble vitamins, help with hormone reactions, and a number of other supportive roles.

Not all fats are created equal, and it is still necessary to use fats in moderation due to their high calorie content. Small amounts of polyunsaturated fats, like olive oil and avocado keep the body running like a well-oiled machine. However, saturated animal fats like lard and butter should be eaten much less often, as they are transported through the blood in cholesterol. Excess saturated fat increases cholesterol, and blocks arteries.

When the body doesn't have enough energy coming in through the diet and fat stores have been depleted, it will begin breaking down muscle as a last resort. Unfortunately, vital organs, including the heart are made of muscle, and severe medical conditions can occur. Not to worry, this would only happen during times of famine, where no food source is available, and the body begins wasting away.

Good nutrition begins with a well rounded variety of all of these foods on a daily basis. Choose lean proteins like chicken breast, eggs, steak or pork chops, along with plant-based proteins like edamame and black beans to make up about 25% of your daily calories. A variety of non-starchy, low carb vegetables should be incorporated as well, and should make up about 50% of your daily plate. Think about having a big mixed vegetable salad with a palm-size portion of protein mixed in. Fats should be used in moderation, including about a teaspoon per meal, but could possibly be more depending on your calorie needs. This could be your salad dressing or a pad of butter on a roll.

Don't forget about carbohydrates either. While they should be consumed in moderation, they are the body's preferred source of fuel, and including them will make you feel satisfied after a meal. Include at least a ½ cup serving of rice or potato, or 1 tablespoon of dried fruit to your salad to balance it out.

Make sure to limit foods that may be detrimental to your health, like alcohol and caffeine, as well as highly processed foods like cookies and crackers. These foods can all hinder your metabolism and work against your good health. Limit alcohol to one drink per day or less, and limit caffeine to 200mg per day, about 1 cup as well. When it comes to snacks, the more refined the sugar is, the more it will affect your metabolism. Sugars that are already broken down skip the digestion process and immediately trigger the release of insulin, the hormone responsible for storing the sugars as fat. Spikes and dips in insulin create an unstable environment, and eventually lead to the development of diabetes.

If you feel you may not be getting enough nutrients from food, and you are off balance, do your best to correct your diet using real foods. Unfortunately, busy lifestyles often make it difficult to plan meals that fit all of your needs. In these cases, the use of supplements can be helpful to keep the balance. Try protein shakes to add protein on the go. Pair with a piece of fruit for a complete meal.

In general, the use of supplements to enhance health is not necessary, and can be a waste of time and resources. Vitamin and mineral supplements should only be used with people who have a legitimate deficiency, and their health has quickly become effected. The increase in specific nutrients can correct the deficiency, but adding more of any nutrient than is required doesn't do much to increase performance, and could potentially be harmful in large doses.

Now that you have a good idea what a basic diet should look like, it is time to tailor your plan to optimally work with your current exercise regimen. The following chapters will examine the ratio of macronutrients that will be beneficial to different training scenarios, as well as discuss the importance of timing of meals for maximum energy while avoiding gastrointestinal distress. Use the recommendations to alter your plan until you find something that works best for you.

Chapter 5: Nutrition for Endurance Training

Endurance training, at its core, requires the body to use just about all of its muscles, including the heart, as well as the lungs to increase intake of oxygen, all for extended periods of time. Have you have ever tried to start a running routine after a long stretch of sedentary behavior? If so, then you know that overdoing it makes your muscles sore, your heart beat out of your chest, and your lungs hurt.

While your stamina will only begin to increase with practice, it is necessary to provide your body with the energy it requires to support the increased needs of the heart, lungs and muscles. In this chapter, we will look at the classic endurance subject, the distance runner. This person has trained for months, and is ready to run a marathon. How can they eat to provide energy to run 26.2 miles without extreme exhaustion?

During training, the runner will need to eat the standard diet we already discussed. They will still need a variety of carbohydrates, proteins and fats. On long training days, the most important thing will be recovery after the long workout. The muscles will be depleted, so protein will be needed after the workout, as well as a good serving of carbohydrates to replenish used stores.

In general, a higher carbohydrate ratio can be used in the daily diet to support distance running. As explained before, carbohydrate can be used for immediate energy. A good deal is stored as glycogen in the liver before it is turned to fat for storage, so keeping the liver stores up will provide readily available energy, enough for a day or two without food. This should be enough to sustain the body during training.

After a workout, eat a meal that is high in both protein and carbs, within about an hour. If the protein is not immediately available for the repair of muscle, lactic acid builds up in the muscle, which causes them to be sore. Swiftly providing fuel will decrease this fatigue, weakness and soreness.

With endurance exercise, it is important to be light on your feet. That is, the more you weigh, the more your muscles have to work to move you. When feeding yourself, make sure to stay within your calorie limits appropriate for your activity level, to avoid excess fat storage and weight. The more streamlined you can be, the less weight the body needs to move, and the longer your glycogen stores will last. This will result in increased performance and stamina.

While there are a number of supplements available that boast increased performance with exercise, don't get carried away. The most important thing is getting a multitude of nutrients from the diet, and that should really be enough. Managing timing of meals and focusing on nutrients from real food is more effective than any supplement will ever be.

Use the following basic training schedule to start tailoring your intake with your exercise regimen:

Basic training schedule: (total calorie amounts will vary)

- **6am:** Wake
- **Breakfast by 7am** (within 1 hour of waking). Should consist of protein and a good dose of carbohydrate. On a race day or heavy workout day, make sure to eat light, utilizing non-fibrous carbs like toast or sweet potato to avoid GI distress. Vegetables or fruits may have too much fiber.
- **8am:** Workout 1-2 hours, cardio based.
- **10am:** Snack-pair protein with carbohydrate, 1:1 ratio. Try a fruit and nut combo for a good mix of carb, protein and fat. Be sure to replenish water as well.
- **12pm:** Lunch-should consist of a large plate of non-starchy vegetables, 20g protein plus 1-2 servings of carbohydrate, like a whole sweet potato.
- **3pm:** Snack-pair protein with carbohydrate, 1:1 ratio. Try a banana and scoop of peanut butter for a quick snack.
- **6pm:** Dinner-should model lunch, focusing on vegetables and protein, with a small dose of carbohydrates.
- **9pm:** have another small snack should you not go to sleep within 3 hours of dinner.

Chapter 6: Preparing for race day

Gearing up for race day changes the scenario a bit. You often hear of runners carb loading the day before the race, often holding pasta dinners for athletes the night before the race. The idea is to load the body with carbs to top off their liver glycogen stores, so that they will have as much immediate energy available as possible. Once those stores are gone, the body will begin to fatigue, as the metabolism must take time to change to using fat for energy, a more laborious, slow process. Keeping the tank topped off ensures longer stretches of good energy before "hitting the wall" as they say.

The morning of the race, it is important to fuel the body without weighing it down. Having a big breakfast before a race will give you the energy you need, but will also make you feel heavy and sluggish, decreasing performance. Avoid high fiber foods like vegetables that can cause GI distress, and focus on foods that provide a lot of carb in a small package so it does not weigh you down. Have a nutrient packed meal, like eggs and toast at least an hour before the race, so that there is time for a bowel movement if necessary. Avoid caffeine, as this can cause GI distress as well.

The goal during the race is to intermittently fuel the body with more carbs to avoid letting the tank run dry. Runners often stop off for water or electrolyte drinks during the race, but have also begun to replenish fuel as well. Eating carbs to replenish has shown to be the best way to maintain energy to finish the race. The problem with eating during a race is the possibility of gastrointestinal distress.

When the body is under stress, in this case, intense exercise, it uses all of its energy to support the activity, and temporarily shuts down systems like the stomach and intestines to save energy. As food is flushed into the resting GI tract, flushing can occur, pushing water into the belly, causing pain, discomfort and the urge to have a bowel movement, nothing you want to happen during a race. The more food you put in, the worse the symptoms will be.

The goal becomes giving the body the carbs it needs in a small package, so that the fuel gets in without taxing the body. Things like high-sugar chocolate milk in small doses is sometimes used, but more technically advanced products have been developed specifically made for runners. Think high-carb juice boxes for adults. While doing intense exercise, the body's glycogen stores last about 90 minutes, requiring a boost at least twice during a marathon run. Plan your run accordingly, staying ahead of glycogen store depletion to better your time.

The only way to increase endurance and speed with running, or any endurance exercise, is to practice. This is how you build up muscle strength and continually support the muscles with fuel and protein for recovery. While it is important to push your limits during training, you are breaking down muscle tissue in the process, and it becomes vital to provide the protein required to repair that damage in a timely manner. If the body has the amino acids it needs, it will not only repair the damage, it will build up the muschel to be able to withstand that level of training again. Your body loves to continually improve itself to be ready next time.

Physiologically speaking, the body does not know the difference between running a marathon and running away from a prehistoric predator. You may have escaped the last training session (or saber-toothed tiger), but next time might not be so lucky, so it is better to prep the muscles for the next life-threatening situation.

Race day variation:
Carb loading should be done the day before, not the morning of. Dinner the night before should be carb based, including rice or pasta with the normal amount of protein and vegetables. Be sure not to overstuff yourself, as this may make you sluggish the following day. To increase the amount of carbs, decrease the serving of vegetables to make room.

Make sure to hydrate as well, as it is never good to start a race dehydrated. Increase total water content for the entire day before. Never before bed, as you will likely not get a good night sleep if you need to keep getting up.

The morning of the race, have a small meal consisting mainly of carbs to top off carb stores. Avoid fibrous foods, sticking to carbs from bread or banana in small doses. Be sure not to overstuff yourself.

Chapter 7: Nutrition for Weight Training

Gaining muscle primarily requires hard work. No nutrition plan or supplement will ever build muscle if you are not working them out. Muscle can only be gained by working them, causing them to be rebuilt better and stronger for next time.

Continually push yourself during workouts by increasing weight and number of reps as appropriate. Consult with a training coach to determine what the best, safest workout is for you, as overstraining muscles and pushing yourself too hard will lead to injuries of muscles, joints and tendons. This is the quickest and easiest way to ruin all of your progress.

From a nutritional standpoint, we must focus on the repair and rebuild of muscles after a workout. Unlike endurance training, it really isn't necessary to carb load, or even load up on protein before working out, as long as you have eaten consistently throughout the day. In general, eating within an hour of waking, then every 3-4 hours throughout the day after will provide more than enough energy to make it through your workout. Muscle repair does not happen until the body is at rest, so loading up on protein before a workout doesn't do much.

A sufficient diet for muscle building requires more protein than the average diet. Your diet should include a minimum of 0.8g/kg of protein per day. For example, a 200 pound person would require a minimum of 72g of protein per day to replenish muscle stores. An ounce of animal protein contains about 7g of protein, so about 10oz of meat per day minimum is required. Many people ask whether it is possible to gain muscle on a vegetarian or vegan diet. The answer is yes, it is possible, but because plant-based products provide less protein per ounce than meat, it will take much more. In fact, it would take about 5 cups of beans per day to get the same amount of protein. Vegan protein powders made from pea and rice proteins can be used to supplement, but it will still take a number of heavy shakes daily to have the same effect. Depending on how your stomach reacts to large amounts of food, this may or may not be a plausible option.

Also, plant-based proteins aren't complete proteins, leading to slower muscle recovery, as they are lacking some of the essential amino acids needed for optimal recovery. For better, faster results, animal based proteins are the way to go, but also must come from lean sources like chicken breast, that do not have excess fat.

Chapter 8: After weight training workout

After a workout, it is important to flood the system with protein in order for quick recovery of muscles. When muscles are working, they require oxygen to facilitate the process of providing the energy required. When oxygen isn't available, muscles produce lactate to make energy, which produces lactic acid as a byproduct.

Lactic acid is responsible for muscle soreness and weakness after a workout. It is normal to feel a bit shaky or weak immediately after a workout as your muscles are exhausted. This is how you know the muscle was truly worked. The presence of this lactic acid stimulates the repair process.

Drinking plenty of water during and after exercise helps neutralize the acid and prevent problems with excess lactic acid buildup that can be harmful to the body.

The weight trainer's diet isn't simply about protein. In fact, too much protein in the diet will be converted to fat if it cannot be immediately used. It is important for weight lifters to stay within an appropriate calorie level for their activity, the same as for endurance training.

Many weight lifters make the mistake of focusing solely on lifting weights, however, it is important to be well rounded, working on cardio training as well. This is especially important to keep fat stores in check. As you remember, excess calories get stored as fat, and the only way to use them is with aerobic exercise. Those muscles cannot be seen if they are covered with a layer of fat.

Start your workout routine with 15-20 minutes of cardio to burn some fat. There are lots of workouts that involve HIIT, or high intensity interval training, which alternates cardio and weight training for a maximum calorie burn. If you have excess fat to burn, this is a great method to do that, while also building muscle. Also, increasing oxygen flow in the body gives your muscles the ability to make energy with that oxygen. The more oxygen can be used, the less lactate is required, lessening the buildup of lactic acid. Using aerobics while weight training can lessen these effects. Doing a bit of cardio also loosens muscles and joints, decreasing the chances of injuries during your workout.

Use the following daily training template to begin tailoring good nutrition to your workout schedule.

Basic training schedule: (total calorie amounts will vary)
- **6am:** Wake
- **Breakfast by 7am** (within 1 hour of waking). Should consist of at least 14g protein, equivalent to 2 eggs, as well as carbohydrate, and fat. Limit fat to ¼ avocado on the eggs or 1 tsp butter on the toast.
- **8am:** Workout x2 hours
- **10am:** Protein shake for recovery within 1 hour of workout. Should provide 20g protein.

- **12pm:** Lunch-should consist of a large plate of non-starchy vegetables, 20g protein plus 1-2 servings of carbohydrate, like a whole sweet potato.
- **3pm:** Snack-pair protein with carbohydrate, 1:1 ratio. Try a banana and scoop of peanut butter for a quick snack.
- **6pm:** Dinner-should model lunch, focusing on vegetables and protein, with a small dose of carbohydrates.
- **9pm:** have another small snack should you not go to sleep within 3 hours of dinner.

Certain micronutrients should be avoided during weight training as well. This is especially important should you be training for a body building competition. Sodium from food attracts water in the body. As sodium enters the diet, water follows, and will stay where the salt is until it gets flushed out. Reducing sodium reduces the buildup of water, which gives more definition to muscles.

Conclusion

Thank for making it through to the end of *Sports Nutrition: The Base Manual For Obtaining Maximum Performance.* I truly hope it was informative and able to provide you with all of the tools you need to achieve your goals of increased performance and stamina during your exercise routine.

The next step is to implement some of these changes, and experiment with different variations in your eating program in order to find out what is best for you. Proper ratios of macronutrients and meal timing can be variable person to person. So, if you find that a specific part of the plan hinders your progress, just adapt it to your personal needs.

Keep a journal of your food choices, meal timing and training schedule to find trends between food, your performance and any distress of your gastrointestinal system.

ALKALINE WATER

CHANGE YOUR WORLD BY BUILDING THE HEALTHY LIFESTYLE

"Drinking water is essential to a healthy lifestyle."

–Stephen Curry

TABLE OF CONTENTS

INTRODUCTION

"Water is life, and clean water means health."
–Audrey Hepburn

In their own way, every person is in search of a healthier life, through diet, exercise, supplements, and lifestyle changes. We alter how often we exercise, how we exercise, what we eat, what we drink, what supplements we take, or such things like whether we smoke or not. Humans have been obsessed with longevity and health as long as our race has been here. Through myths from almost four centuries ago, for instance, everyone followed the trail of the Fountain of Youth, and we have dedicated books, movies, and stories to the elusive search for eternal life. We spend millions of dollars every year on exercise programs, bottled water, and supplements, among other things, in order to look younger and feel better.

A basic building block of life, water is essential for every living organism on the planet. We can simply drink from our taps to satisfy our thirst, or we can make the best of what we put into our bodies and ensure that every sip boosts our health. Water, taken in an alkaline form, can serve many purposes aside from simple hydration inside the human body. These purposes include:

- Reducing cholesterol
- Reducing inflammation
- Improving the immune system
- Helping with weight loss
- Boosting energy
- And more!

With the huge number of options on the market when it comes to the types of bottled water – distilled, purified, ionized, sparkling, mineral, flavored – not to mention the simple decision of whether to spend $1.25 per day to buy a bottle water or to fill up your own glass carafe right from your own tap, most people tend to choose the purchased bottled water as the best option. But that might not always be the best choice. We are all looking for the healthiest alternative and, as is always the case, it pays to be informed. Test your tap water, test your favorite bottled water – see which ones are the best ones to put in your mouth, not only for its flavor but also for the benefits that it can provide you on a basic cellular level.

For every system, there is a delicate balance between acid and alkaline. Our cells, our organs, our bodies work best when their own necessary pH balance is maintained. We should all do what we can to help those systems work more efficiently. If we put the right ingredients into the engine, then we can get the best results. That includes both the best food and water that are available. If your research leads you to follow an alkaline approach, there are a number of healthy options. To get to those alkaline ingredients, there are a number of paths that allow us to choose the best options to make the most of the benefits.

For example, sometimes the tap water that we drink falls within alkaline levels, and sometimes we have to treat the water we have or buy water that is within acceptable ranges. Processed foods should be avoided, and more raw fruits and vegetables should be introduced into our daily intake. The alkaline water should be rich with alkalizing compounds such as silica, potassium, magnesium, bicarbonate, and calcium. By ionizing the water and ensuring it is alkaline, the health benefits are the highest it could be, which would do the best inside the body. This type of water introduces negative ions into the system, and those negative ions can help put a stop to diseases.

If you aren't lucky enough to live in a city that has alkaline water coming from the taps, then there are a number of devices on the market that can be purchased that can help you convert ordinary water to alkaline, ionized or purified water. There are a host of different types of equipment and machines on the market that can convert the water into the best version of itself: pitcher filters, reverse osmosis, water ionizers (countertop and in-cabinet), and water distillers – something to fit every budget and every preferred approach to good health.

With the vast array of knowledge at our fingertips and the ability to order what we need online, the supplies showing up right on our doorstep, and with our never-ending search for good health, there is no longer an excuse to take anything less than the best approach to the best health that we can have.

Chapter 1:
WHAT IS ALKALINE WATER?

"Water is the most important thing you put in your body, but not all water is equal."
–Dr. Henri Coanda

As frail human beings, we are constantly in search of something that will improve our health, increase our beauty, and provide us with a long and healthy life. We change our diets, our exercise routines, and we travel the world in search of other benefits. And although our search may lead us far and wide, an everyday benefit may be as close as our sinks and refrigerators.

One of the staples of many of the health industries is water: everyone knows that water is a basic element of a healthy lifestyle. However, there are always ways we can improve even the best of approaches. The theory of how much water the human body needs varies greatly depending on your school of thought. Some believe that most people need to drink at least eight 8-oz glasses of water per day.

Other health experts believe that it is a more complicated formula for body weight and activity level. This formula involves taking a person's body weight, multiplying it by two-thirds, and then adjusting the total amount depending on the person's activity level. In other words, if you are a fairly active person who exercises approximately 30 minutes per day, another 12 oz of water should be added to the total water intake. In addition, drinking approximately 2 cups of water before meals can help a person lose 5 pounds per year by increasing the metabolic rate and tricking our brains into thinking we are full before we are. It takes the brain 20 minutes to catch up with the stomach, so we continue to eat long after we are technically full. By drinking the water shortly before we start eating, we are far more likely to stop eating with less food in our stomach. And, although any type of water can hydrate, alkaline water is better at it and may have some other benefits as well.

Some research shows that alkaline water can:

- Balance the ratio of beneficial minerals
- Boost the immune system
- Boost vitamin absorption
- Decrease leptins
- Flush out kidney stones and prevent their recurrence
- Improve skin condition and complexion
- Improve energy levels
- Improve the production of human growth hormones

- Lower chronic pain and inflammation
- Lower the risk of hypertension and stroke
- Lower the risk of osteoporosis
- Maintain a healthy weight by flushing out toxins
- Help protect against cancer
- Promote better digestion (as acid interferes with the normal digestion process)
- Protect against bad cholesterol (can possibly even convert bad to good)
- Protect bone density
- Protect muscle mass
- Slow the aging process
- Support weight loss (by flushing toxins out of system)

By ionizing the water, our bodies can more easily absorb hydration as this water contains smaller molecules. Ionizing the water also gives the calcium and magnesium a negative charge which helps the body to recognize them as more absorbable. In addition, the negative charge of the extra electron acts as a natural antioxidant and may have the potential to neutralize free radicals within the body.

However, there is a difference between naturally alkaline water and water that is created through an artificial process. With two samples of water, each at a pH rating of 9.0 and both being alkaline, if one occurs naturally from an underground spring and one has come out of an electronic water ionizer, there will be fundamental differences. The naturally occurring water with the higher pH may have an abundance of minerals present in the water as well. The presence of those minerals in the alkaline water is what can boost the benefits of alkaline water to the next step. Fortunately, some tap waters that are available to the public test positively for alkalinity, thereby giving consumers the benefits of alkaline water which is packed full of minerals that the human body can use.

Since ionized/alkaline water contains negative ions, it alters the human system. Biological aging is an ongoing process whereby a stream of positive ions begins to eat away at our health until we finally fall prey to a variety of diseases. If you can introduce negative ions to the system and have them begin to outweigh the positive, your health can improve. One way to do that is to eat raw foods, and another is to drink ionized/alkaline water.

Some critics argue that alkaline water must occur naturally to be the most beneficial for consumption. The pH of the water should match the mineral content; if the pH doesn't match the minerals, the pH of the water will then become unstable. Some critics also state that if water is artificially altered, the water will quickly revert back to the pH in keeping with its natural mineral content. By consuming any treated water with an unstable/artificial pH, we may, in fact, be negatively affecting our health as it may cause nervous tension, a compromised immune system, and possible injury to cardiac tissues. This indicates that the only manner alkaline water can be beneficial would be when it is a naturally occurring substance.

Pure water, known as ionic water, is the best choice, comprising essential minerals but managing to remove harmful contaminants such as lead, aluminum, bacteria, chlorine hormones, pesticides, and nitrates. Alkaline water is water that has been chemically or fundamentally altered, and synthetic materials may be added to it. Alkaline ionized water is water created by electrolysis using equipment. The alkaline water ionizer contains dissolved hydrogen gas, also referred to as diatomic or molecular hydrogen. The hydrogen ion that is not bound to a water molecule makes the ion available to the body as an antioxidant. This hydrogen can trap toxic free radicals and convert them to water, allowing them to be eliminated from the body. There have been almost 400 articles and over 30 studies conducted on humans regarding the benefits of hydrogen on the system. This can be one of the best uses of water – as a natural antioxidant that removes free radicals from the body.

Some advocates of alkaline water indicate that the benefit of the water lies not as much in the pH rating but in the amount of dissolved hydrogen. This extra hydrogen is processed in the body as an antioxidant. Hydrogen gas, a substance found naturally in the body, has been the subject of numerous studies over the years and is thought to be therapeutic for the majority of human organs and a treatment for over 100 diseases. However, the hydrogen in water is very temperate as hydrogen will completely evaporate within 24 hours. Therefore, alkaline water created to be ionized water should be consumed within 24 hours to get the most benefits from it. This school of thought indicates that none of the alkaline ionized water that is pre-bottled would be beneficial to anyone's health.

The start of the alkaline water industry boils down to the search of the human race for something that will improve health and help us stay young as long as possible. Around the world, there are several locations where the population seems to enjoy the fruits of a longer life and lower potential for disease. Those places inspired an entire industry trying to replicate the life-affirming molecules that can be found in the water. These regions are called blue zones, and one of the most famous of those, the Hunza Valley found in the Himalayas, inspired the life-long search of two men, Dr. Henri Coanda and Patrick Flanagan, to try to discover and replicate those benefits. These investigations may be one of the things that led to the use of alkaline water to improve health and longevity.

Chapter 2:
WHERE CAN YOU GET ALKALINE WATER?

"Nothing is softer or more flexible than water, yet nothing can resist it."
–Lao Tzu

The easiest way to get alkaline water is simply to buy it pre-packaged. However, as indicated earlier, there is a school of thought that believes this type of water is less beneficial as the extra hydrogen is no longer active after the first 24 hours. There are a number of bottled waters on the market that have a pH rate high enough to qualify as alkaline water (above a 7.0 on the pH scale). Those leading brands on the market are:

- Absopure
- Acqua Panna
- Crystal Geyser
- Essentia
- Eternal
- Evamor
- Evian
- Fiji
- JUST water
- Real Water
- Resource (Nestle)
- Super Chill
- Volvic
- Zephyrhills

All of the above have a pH rating that's more alkaline, or higher than 7.0 (neutral rating). The following table describes each brand with a slightly more detailed description of the rating, source, ownership, minerals, and other known information. Since the available information for each one cannot be standardized (i.e., source, processing, pH level, etc.), the amount and type of information per brand may vary greatly.

Brand of Water	Type of Water	Details	Where to Buy
Absopure	Absopure Plus – vapor distilled water with electrolytes added	The company was established in 1908; provides both home delivery and bottled water on the market; first company to recycle their own bottles; located in mid-western U.S.	Kroger Walmart Home delivery Amazon
Acqua Panna	Mineral spring water	Available from Tuscany; underground spring water that takes 13 years to flow from the aquifer to the surface at extremely low temperature	Amazon Walmart Publix
Crystal Geyser	Alpine spring water – naturally occurring electrolytes and minerals; not filtered or treated	Only major U.S. bottled water that is collected directly from an authentic natural spring; owned by CG Roxanne LLC and established in 1990; involved in a number of environmental partnerships	Walgreens Target Amazon DollarTree Kroger
Essentia	Ionized alkaline water; pH rating of 9.5; contains trace amounts of electrolytes	Filtered and treated water (proprietary ionization process), microfiltration, reverse osmosis, and UV exposure makes it 99.9% pure; headquartered in Washington, but available across the country	Walmart CVS Amazon Bi-Lo Publix Kroger

Brand of Water	Type of Water	Details	Where to Buy
Eternal	Alkaline spring water; natural electrolytes, not artificially treated or filtered	Based in Tennessee, New York, and California	Walmart Kroger Publix Amazon
Evamor	High alkaline artesian water; pH fluctuates between 8.8 and 9.1; natural, not filtered or processed; contains minerals	Originates in the U.S.	Health stores Amazon
Evian	Natural mineral water; pH at 7.2; naturally filtered and contains the minerals sodium potassium, calcium, magnesium, bicarbonates, sulfates, and silicates	Sourced from the Alps	Amazon Walmart Publix Kroger
Fiji	Natural artesian; filtered through lava rock	Company founded in 1996; number one imported bottled water in the U.S. and distributed to over 60 countries around the world	Amazon Walmart Kroger Publix
JUST Water	Spring water	Paper-based bottle and the cap made from sugarcane; sourced from Glens Falls watershed	Kroger Amazon

Brand of Water	Type of Water	Details	Where to Buy
Real Water	Alkalized water; pH 8.0	Uses a proprietary E2 Technology which means it can maintain a stable negative ionization; owned by Affinity Lifestyles; both home delivery and bottled	Health food stores Whole Foods Amazon
Resource	Spring water; contains natural electrolytes and minerals	Nestlé is the parent company; bottles are 100% recycled plastic	Walmart Amazon
Volvic	Natural spring water; natural balance of electrolytes and minerals; minerals in the water include calcium, sulfates, magnesium, potassium, bicarbonate, silica, and chlorides	Available since 1958, top-selling brand in France, Germany, UK, Japan, and Ireland; company part of the Danone Group (distributed in the U.S. by Brands Within Reach, LLC); originates in France; water source is about 90 meters below the surface – only sees sunlight when it is bottled	Amazon Walmart Publix
Zephyrhills	Natural spring water; carbonated after by a process; ten-step filtration/quality process after it is sourced	Bottled in Florida; spring found in 1910; in 1964, the water company starts; five spring sources in a town known as "The City of Pure Water"	Walmart Target CVS Amazon

A number of these brands are available through major retail chains, such as Walmart, Publix, Target, and Fresh Market, while others must be ordered online through Amazon or other specialty shops and health food stores. Still, others are only available regionally, and you may have to travel to find what you need.

If you don't wish to purchase, you can make your own alkaline water at home naturally, or you can use any number of specialty devices. Either of these processes is relatively easy; you can produce the water using simple kitchen ingredients, or you can buy a number of devices that let you convert your water into alkaline water (e.g., reverse osmosis pitchers, countertop ionizers). See the following section for a complete list of the types of home systems that can produce quality alkaline water and how they each work.

Chapter 3:
HOW DO YOU MAKE ALKALINE WATER?

"Water is the driving force of all nature."
–Leonardo da Vinci

There are a number of at-home devices that can be used to produce beneficial alkaline and ionized water. The approach depends mostly on the amount of money you want to invest and the type of process that you prefer. Filtration systems for individual and household water supplies exist, and they can convert water for the entire house's use or just for the supply you keep in the refrigerator. Some can transform your water into alkaline, and some just remove the contaminants and other toxins to ensure that your water is as healthy as it can be.

Water Ionizer

In a water ionizer, a unit is attached to a faucet, and the water is electrically enhanced (ionized) by running the water over positive and negative electrodes in a process known as electrolysis. Tap water is processed over plates, typically platinum and titanium, which causes the exchange of ions. This separates the water into alkaline and acid. The alkalized water makes up about 70% of the refined water. The acidic water that is the remaining 30% is very good at killing bacteria. It can be used as a wash for various parts of the body or for fruits and vegetables. A faucet-mounted system (which typically costs $20-30) is easy to install but has a slow water flow and may not fit on the faucet you currently have installed. A countertop filter ($100-1000) will filter a larger quantity of water but would require modifications in your plumbing which could also potentially require professional assistance. This type of filer is also more likely to clog, and it will clutter your countertops. For those with limited kitchen space, this could be an issue.

Pitcher Filter

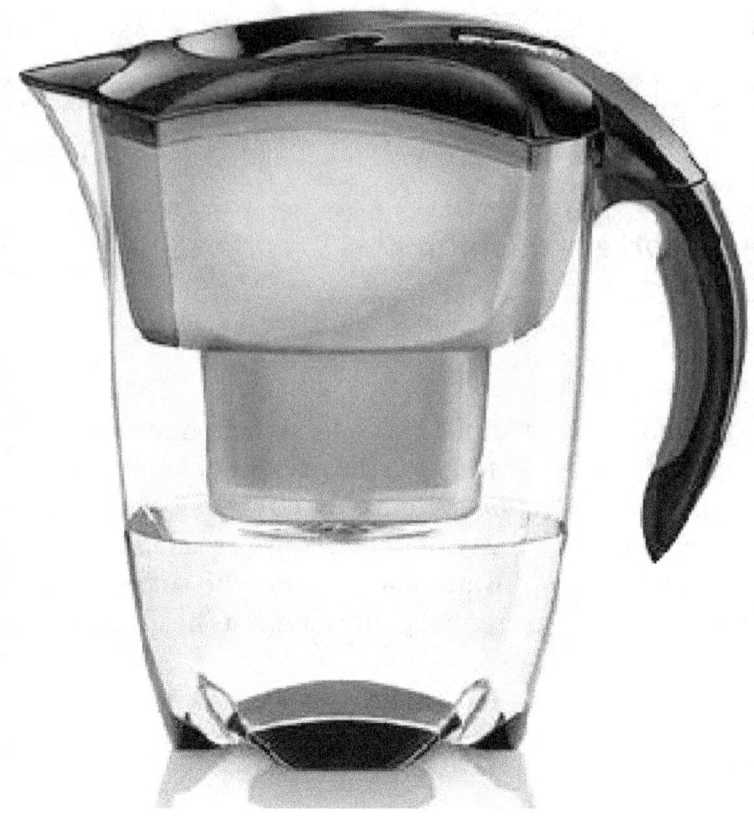

This is cheaper than an electric system. To use it, you pour the water into the pitcher and wait for about 3-5 minutes. The water in the filter passes through a series of filters and sits in a pool of alkalizing minerals. Ensure that the purchased pitcher indicates that it meets with NSF certification (a non-profit testing lab that develops standards for the industry) which will ensure that the water processed meets alkaline standards. A pitcher (or carafe) water filter averages $20-70 to purchase at major retailers. They produce a smaller amount of water, take a longer time to process, and have a short filter life, but they are affordable and easy to refrigerate.

Reverse Osmosis Filter

This type of system uses a hyper-filter to capture more elements than regular water filters. Since the membrane is so fine, this raises the quality of the filtration performed. A reverse osmosis filter (typically costing $150-1800) will probably require you to sacrifice some cabinet space in the kitchen as well as to periodically replace the membranes and filters. It will also produce 3-5 gallons of wastewater while generating alkaline water at a very slow water flow. The filters can sometimes be very expensive to maintain.

Water Distillers

These systems boil the water to remove impurities. Unfortunately, the quality of the output depends greatly on the water that you have to begin with. Some contaminants and chemicals do not boil away, so if they exist before the boil process, they will remain afterward.

Alkaline Drops

There are a number of brands on the market that can be artificially added to any type of water. These drops are available in most health food stores and can be purchased online as well. Although most drops have a basis of distilled or deionized water, they are typically a conglomeration of chemicals or minerals that facilitate an alkaline reaction. These drops involve creating the alkaline water artificially. Some of the drops on the market simply raise the alkaline level of the water and some can add minerals and antioxidants as well. If you are drinking alkaline water as a healthy alternative, you may want to be careful with the additional minerals and additives such as potassium hydroxide, sodium hydroxide, potassium lactate, tri-potassium phosphate, potassium bicarbonate, potassium citrate, magnesium chloride, zinc lactate, sodium selenite, calcium chloride, potassium sorbate, ascorbic acid, niacin, folic acid, and others.

This open can seem less expensive initially, but it can be an ongoing expense as most treatments require 6-8 drops per 8-ounce glass of water, and there are only 100 drops per container. If one container costs approximately $20 and treats approximately 16 glasses of water and you are drinking the recommended amount of water per day (8 glasses), then the contents would only last 2 days. Thus, while the drops are easier to use, it maybe not be the best option for everyone. Make sure to follow the directions on the bottle as each one has specific requirements. When added to water, these substances release oxygen in the body which assists in fixing the biochemical balance. These can also come in powder form which may contain a mixture of other alkaline materials such as calcium, iron, manganese, potassium, or magnesium. Usage will vary from company to company, and instructions from the package should be followed explicitly.

Infrared Filter

This type uses an ultraviolet (UV) light to destroy viruses and bacteria. These systems reduce the lead contaminants and chloride but do not reduce the beneficial minerals found in water. Typically, they are installed where the water enters your house (on the incoming line), so a dedicated faucet is not needed. They are not as effective as a reverse osmosis system in removing contaminants, but they also do not remove the minerals that are needed to make water healthy. These will not affect the pH rating of water; while it will not make water more alkaline, however, it will make it more pure.

If you don't want to use a device or create your alkaline water artificially, you can make your own homemade version of alkaline water with a few simple ingredients you can find at your local grocery store or in your kitchen. To get started, you'll need:

- A one-gallon glass container (preferably with a lid)

- A gallon of distilled or purified water
- Baking soda
- pH test strips (or an electronic pH meter)
- Sea salt
- Coral calcium powder
- Lemon
- Knife, bowl, and measuring cup

To make the water:

1. Pour some of the distilled or purified water into your glass container.

2. Add one teaspoon of baking soda, coral calcium, and sea salt.

3. Roll the lemon on a countertop and cut in half. Juice the lemon, removing seeds.

4. Add the lemon juice into the water. Shake the container to combine.

5. Add the remaining distilled or purified water to this concentrated mixture.

6. Let at least 1-2 inches of air remain at the top of the container.

7. Use the pH strips (or pH meter) to test the water. If you are at 8-9 on the pH scale, then the water is ready for consumption; if not, add more baking soda and shake again to ensure it is combined. Repeat tests again until you achieve the desired effects.

Chapter 4:
IS ALKALINE WATER HEALTHY?

"If there is magic on this planet, it is contained in water."
–Loren Eiseley

Hydration is a watch-word with a lot of diet and exercise programs, and alkaline water is composed of water molecules that are much smaller and more readily absorbed by your cells. Thus, it makes the water you do ingest that much more easily used by the cells that need it. So the question must be focused on the approach of increasing the alkaline in your body. As with anything else, there are two sides to the argument. Some fields of thought believe that diseases and cancer can only exist in an acidic state; therefore, if you increase the alkaline levels of your body, then disease and cancer cannot exist. This then reduces your risks of ever developing these types of disease.

THE PROS

However, each organ system in the human body has a specific pH range that may affect the performance and efficiency of the system. If you are experiencing symptoms, the first and smartest step may be to get tested to find out why the system is not functioning properly. For example, because of increased CO_2 deposition, the pH of the ocean has dropped from 8.2 to 8.1. That may seem like a small change, but this has affected the very existence of some sea life.

Studies have been conducted since the early 1950s regarding the benefit of alkaline water (see section on the history of alkaline water). A study done in 2012 showed how drinking water with a pH of 8.8 may help reduce the levels of pepsin, which is the main enzyme that causes acid reflux. Each organ system in the human body has an optimum level of pH at which they function. Any imbalance in the functioning pH levels can lead to malfunctions such as chronic low-grade metabolic acidosis. This can become significant and may lead to metabolic imbalances like kidney stones, bone health issues (reduced mineral density), loss of muscle mass, and risk of certain chronic diseases (diabetes, high blood pressure). A similar study watched 100 people who were involved in exercising and monitored the effect of alkaline water. The results showed that the alkaline water reduced the viscosity of the blood, which allowed the blood to more easily flow through the body, delivering oxygen to the organs and cells in a more efficient manner.

Proponents of the alkaline water approach feel that drinking it will:

- Slow the aging process

- Regulate your body's pH levels
- Help with colon cleansing (flushing toxins from the system)
- Prevent chronic disease
- Reduce high blood pressure
- Help in lowering dangerous cholesterol
- Reduce the risk of diabetes
- Provide cancer resistance
- Assist with weight loss (again flushing toxins from the system)
- Support the hydration and detoxification process

Athletes and those who enjoy exercising may benefit greatly from drinking alkaline water. The water may allow active people to retain more fluid in the cardiovascular system while decreasing their urine output and blood osmolality. High plasma osmolality is associated with the elevated risk of death from a stroke. High osmolality is the efficiency of the process that causes a liquid to pass through the wall of a living cell, equalizing the concentration of the solution on both sides of the membrane. However, intense exercise spurs our muscles to produce more hydrogen ions than our body can efficiently remove. Alkaline water may help alleviate this, which is why the benefits of alkaline water may be more apparent in those that frequently exercise, but the benefits exist for everyone.

Organs deteriorate and disease sets in over time if you don't flush out acidic waste. The most important organs to protect against acidic waste are the kidneys, lungs, and skin. The kidneys regulate acid and alkaline balance in the bloodstream and eliminate solid or fixed acids through urination. One of those substances that are eliminated is potassium. Potassium is one of the key electrolytes utilized by the body. Its role in the body is to regulate water balance, regulate the acid-base balance in the blood and tissues, control muscle contractions, and control heartbeat, energy metabolism, and biochemical reactions. The body doesn't conserve potassium, however, so it needs to be constantly replenished. For this reason, fluids that are high in electrolytes are very beneficial to the human body. Electrolytes are the smallest chemicals important to the body, and they include:

- Sodium
- Potassium
- Calcium
- Magnesium
- Bicarbonate

Specialized kidney cells monitor the amount of sodium, potassium, and water. Alkaline water is beneficial in assisting the kidney to keep functioning at optimum health limits. The balance of those electrolytes controls specific processes, such as:

- Allowing cells to generate energy
- Maintaining the stability of cell walls
- Assisting in the function of most cells
- Generating electricity
- Contracting muscles
- Moving water and fluids through the body

Alkaline with negative ions may benefit your cholesterol levels as well. Good cholesterol has electrons; bad cholesterol has lost its electrons and has oxidized. That means that the plaque that shows up in the arteries is cholesterol that has oxidized. Bathing the bad cholesterol in electrons will convert it back into good cholesterol – including the plaque. This makes hydrogen and the alkaline water that is laden with it, very beneficial to heart health.

On the other side of the argument are those that don't support the idea that alkaline water is beneficial at all or is beneficial simply because it is alkaline. Dead water or water that has been filtered and processed until all of the contaminants are no longer present, sometimes crosses the line to where there are no longer any beneficial minerals present either. When alkaline water occurs in nature, typically it has run through a series of porous rocks, and that process is all that it takes for a water to have an alkaline pH.

THE CONS

Most pH systems in the body are internally regulated. This means that outside forces cannot chemically alter the pH levels of blood, plasma, or other body fluids. When the human body has excess acid, it expels it through sweat, urine, and breathing. This includes any effect that the alkaline might have on stomach acid. In fact, stomach acid is so acidic that when alkaline water is consumed, even the most alkaline of water doesn't stand a chance. After acidification of the alkaline water, even if the water could somehow manage to retain any alkalinity, it would not affect the pH of the intestines.

Meanwhile, eating too many alkalizing foods may change the pH levels in your intestines, which can lead to an increase in Candida overgrowth. Some researchers feel that almost 70% of all people are affected by Candida. Candida yeast can only evolve into their fungal form and create Candida symptoms when the pH of the intestines is neutral or slightly alkaline. Most of the time, Candida is a fungus that is a microscopic organism that exists harmlessly in the body. However, if the system gets thrown out of balance, the Candida can take over entire systems. Typically, the first system at risk is the digestive system, but Candida infections can manifest in a wide variety of symptoms.

There are very few scientific human health studies performed that can prove drinking alkaline water will have far-reaching health benefits. Yet as much as the benefits of alkaline water may have been overstated, it is not harmful; it just might not be the answer to all your health problems. Plus, in reality, alkaline water can be expensive, not least of which concerning the investment for the initial unit to process water, e.g., the ionizer and the filters that need to be replaced on a regular basis.

Chapter 5:
WHAT ARE pH LEVELS?

"When you're thirsty, and it seems that you could drink the entire ocean, that's faith; when you start to drink and finish only a glass or two, that's science."
–Anton Chekhov

Most of us are familiar with rating pH levels – we did the experiments some time during our stay in school, taking pH test strips and comparing them against the color chart to see what alkaline looks like versus acid. The pH system was founded by a Danish chemist in 1909 and was revised to the modern system, as it currently appears, in 1924. But how does that apply to water and how water can help the human body? Although common, most people don't realize that pH stands for "potential of hydrogen" or, according to other sources, the "power of hydrogen." This has been a work in progress since the early 1900s, and the modern pH scale is a logarithmic scale that is used to specify the acidic or basic nature of a solution that contains water or is water-like. Testing and evaluating the substance measures the activity of the hydrogen in a solution. The logarithm means that there is an exponential increase; i.e., pH 3 is 10 times more acidic than pH 4 and 100 times higher than pH 5.

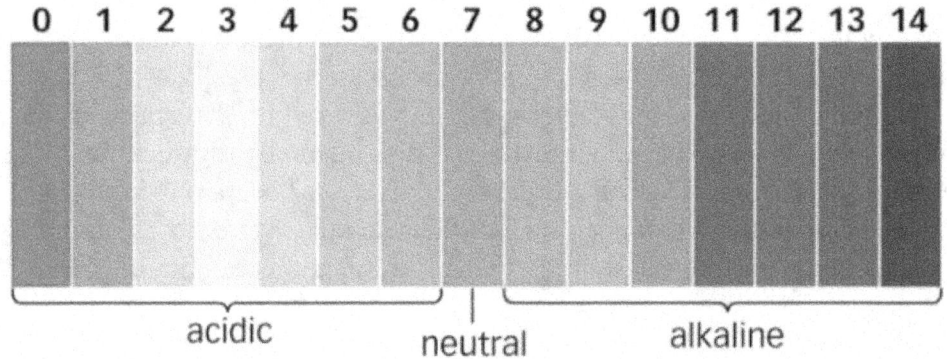

Materials that are highly acid rate a 1 on the pH scale, 7 is neutral, and 14 is completely alkaline. Human systems run the range of substances. Blood pH levels are optimal between 7.35 and 7.45; stomach acid falls at pH 3.5; urine output ranges depending on diet, exercise, and general health. To keep your health at an optimal level, the water of pH between 9 and 10 should be used to keep a healthy body at pH 7.3.

This scale, pictured above, allows anyone to judge the chemical disposition of a substance. According to the scale, strong acids are acids which almost completely dissociate when placed into water, meaning that the molecules break up completely. Weak acids are those that stay mostly undissociated in water. As such, strong acids stay the same but weak acids do not.

Chapter 6:
HOW IS ALKALINE WATER DIFFERENT FROM OTHER WATERS?

"Thousands have lived without love, not one without water."
–W. H. Auden

Alkaline Water

Alkaline water is water with a pH rating above 7, with the best health results coming in at 9-10 on the pH scale. The pH can be the result of natural spring water or tap water. The best way to find out is to test existing water to ensure it's in an alkaline state. If you can ingest alkaline antioxidant water, it is the best type of water for a healthy hydration.

Bottled Water

This is a huge category that encompasses a lot of different waters from several different sources. In 2016, bottled water surpassed soda in sales, at 12.8 billion gallons of total bottled water volume. There is a wide variety of opinions as to the benefit of bottled water. Some opinion is that it is better and more regulated than tap water, while some others say that it is less so.

The source of bottled water varies per company; some are artesian, spring, or tap water. The majority of bottled water companies use extreme filtration (ion-exchange, demineralization, reverse osmosis, distillation, deionization, or any combination of these) to improve the flavor and remove harmful chemicals. However, some of these processes also remove the beneficial minerals as well. Regardless of the source, when water is subjected to extreme filtration, it is proven over and over that you create dead water (no nutritional value).

The FDA considers bottled water as a "good" and sets testing guidelines. It is partially being debated whether the EPA has stricter guidelines or if the FDA guidelines are stringent enough. Bottled water companies are not under the same restraints and guidelines as municipal water sources. Companies do not need to be transparent – they do not have to completely disclose the source of their water or the filtration process they are using.

A number of independent company prepare a "scorecard" for bottled water: Dasani has a pH of 6.4, but the local source is not specified, and their press release on their processes state only that "a special blend of minerals" are added; Aquafina has a pH rating of 6.3 with no information on their source or treatment; Voss has a pH of 7.2, and spring water is stated as their source; SmartWater has a pH of 7.2 and is one of the more transparent companies as to their source and multiple filtration processes. It is important to note that bottled water is not just simply repackaged tap water. If a bottled water plant does use tap water as a source, then there are processes that occur to further treat the water to purify or sterilize the water that is then bottled and sold to the consumer.

Those who cite the shortcomings of bottled water will argue that the regulations are not strict enough and the transparency of the source or treatment of bottled water is lacking. In addition, those same critics would argue that the BPA chemicals in the bottles themselves made the water less of a healthy alternative.

Tap Water

Although bottled water is a billion dollar industry, tap water still outperforms the market on a daily basis. Tap water supplies 1 billion gallons of water every hour of the day. An entire year of bottled water would only supply enough tap water for 9 hours. The quality of tap water varies a great deal from city to city and state to state. Most tap water contains chemicals to kill germs, fungus, and algae. The EPA, which mandates control and quality of tap water, requires water suppliers to provide a Consumer Confidence Report (CCR) for any area providing water to 100,000 people or more. They require water companies to give a detailed account of the source and results of testing, and these results are posted online. Municipal water companies are required to test several times per day – bottled water companies are only required to test one per week (testing for microbes).

Some tap water may contain chemicals that assist in treating bacteria, fungus, and algae. These come with a number of potential side-effects on the human body. Those chemical affects include:

- Benzene: harmful effects on bone marrow, decreases red blood cells, leads to anemia
- Atrazine: may cause low fetal weight; heart, urinary, and limb defects in humans; and slow development of fetuses
- Coliform bacteria: gastro-centric infections (nausea, vomiting, diarrhea, stomach, cramps); none detectible per 100 mL
- Arsenic: carcinogenic (may cause cancer of the bladder, lungs, skin, kidney, nasal passages, liver, and prostate); there can potentially be 10 ppb

However, along with those chemicals, there are also some beneficial minerals in tap water. In addition to these minerals, there are trace elements of copper, zinc, manganese, and iron as well. A daily dose of tap water provides approximately 20% of calcium and magnesium and between 1% and 20% of the following daily recommended intake of minerals, such as:

- Phosphorous: assists with endurance, counteracts fatigue, converts sugar into energy
- Calcium: helps strengthen bones and teeth; helps with blood clotting, cell growth, and hormone production
- Potassium: balances fluids, blood pressure, blood sugar levels, and conduction of nerve impulses
- Magnesium: helps with strong bones, energy, metabolism, and functioning of muscles

Reverse Osmosis Water

The most acidic type of water where the beneficial minerals have also been removed. When this type of water travels through your body, it actually leaches the minerals out of your system. As this is essentially devoid of minerals, it is one of the best types of water to use in small electronics, such as a steam iron, as there will not be any mineral build-up.

Distilled Water

Distilled water is water that is boiled (turned into steam) and then condensed back into liquid, typically in another container. Whatever impurities exist in the water before the distillation process begins can either boil out or remain in the water. This process will remove soluble minerals such as calcium, magnesium, and phosphorus, as well as heavy metals like mercury, lead, and arsenic. But there are some semi-volatile or volatile chemicals that will not be removed by this process (e.g., some pesticides). However, this process will remove any harmful bacteria.

Mineral Water

This is a specialty water that contains not less than 250 parts per million (ppm) total of dissolved solids. The flavor of the water can be greatly changed by the region it derives from, what type of rocks the water flows over, and what the specific mineral content it ends up having. There can exist so much differences that there is now what is known as a Mineral Water Sommelier (although only 100 people in the world could be classified as a professional). The minerals in water can include:

- Calcium carbonate
- Iron
- Sodium
- Magnesium
- Copper
- Manganese
- Lead
- Boron
- Arsenic
- Phosphorous

Water can be hard or soft, also depending upon the minerals found in it. In fact, there are bourbon distilleries in Kentucky that swear their product is the best because of the limestone-filtered water that they start with. Calcium makes water taste milky and smooth, and magnesium can be bitter; sodium tastes salty, of course, and iron gives a metallic taste. As such, changes in percentages and combinations of the minerals can cause an endless variety of flavors. These minerals can even change the hardness of the water and the interaction between the water and materials. For example, water that is hard (too much calcium and magnesium) should not be used to cook beans as the chemical composition will not allow the beans to cook until tender no matter how long they are soaked or cooked.

Spring Water

This is the most recognized and common form of bottled water. This type of water comes from an underground source from which the water flows naturally to the surface. Spring water can be collected only at the source or through a hole which taps directly into the source. This type of water is the most likely to contain minerals from the rocks and soil it is filtered through.

Artesian Water

Artesian is basically another name for spring water, although this refers to a specific type of spring water. This water from underground passes through a layer of rock or clay. Since it is an underground spring, the pressure makes it rise as a water source. When tapped, the water pushes above the level of the rock and clay and sometimes to the surface. Some theories state that artesian water is more pure because the layer of rock and clay impedes the movement of contamination. However, the EPA does not verify this claim.

Purified Water

This classification is for water that has been artificially treated in some manner: distillation, deionization, reverse osmosis, or other processes of purification. This is more of an umbrella term that can cover the more specific types of water such as distilled water, deionized water, or reverse osmosis water. Treatment methods have different outcomes. For instance, deionized water has been treated to remove impurities and minerals have been removed, but bacteria and pathogens have not.

Deionized Water

This is also known as demineralized water and is similar to distilled water. Impurities are eliminated through the removal of mineral ions. The nutrients are also removed, so this type of waterfalls under the category of "purified" water.

Flavored Water

This type of water is artificially flavored and may potentially have vitamins, and minerals added as well. It is typically marketed as a great alternative to sugar-laden soda. However, it is important to do your own research and read the nutritional labels. Some flavored waters can have as much sugar as the sodas they are supposed to be a great substitute for. The process that adds the minerals and nutrients back into the water also adds calories to the water as well.

Sparkling Water

This is simply water that has been treated with carbon dioxide. This treatment can take place with drinking water, mineral water, or spring water. Carbon dioxide is the main ingredient of soda that makes it bubble and fizz. A subcategory of this, tonic water, is sparkling water with quinine added. Tonic water is a typical mixer for alcoholic beverages.

Chapter 7:
WHICH WATERS HAVE HIGHER pH LEVELS AND WHICH HAVE LOWER?

"Life in us is like the water in a river."
–Henry David Thoreau

Municipal or tap water varies from station to station and city to city. Users should perform a pH test on your tap water to see the ratings. You may find out that the tap water in your own city is well within the alkaline range. You also have the option of drinking bottled water, but unfortunately, tests have found the majority of bottled water available on the market are higher in acid than would be preferable for someone who wants to follow an alkaline lifestyle. The easiest way to find out if this is true for you is to test your favorite brand; a pH kit is relatively inexpensive and can be found in most retail stores. Several of the bottled waters on the market is neutral or alkaline. Those include:

Water Name	pH Level	Type of Water	Benefits
Absopure	7.5	Vapor distilled water with electrolytes added	Electrolytes added
Essentia	9.0	Mineral spring water	Alkaline and minerals
Eternal	7.0	Alpine spring water – naturally occurring electrolytes and minerals	Alkaline and electrolytes/minerals
Evamor	8.0	Ionized alkaline water	Alkaline and ionized
Evian	7.0	Alkaline spring water	Alkaline
Fiji	8.0-9.0	High alkaline artesian water; pH fluctuates	Alkaline and minerals

Real Water	8.0	Natural mineral water	Alkaline and minerals
Super Chill	7.5	Natural artesian	alkaline and minerals
Volvic	7.0	Spring water	Alkaline, electrolytes, and minerals
Zephyrhills	7.5	Alkalized water	Alkaline carbonated

The World Health Organization warns against drinking water with a low mineral content, as it will leach minerals from the body to compensate. Pure water has a pH level close to 7; alkaline water would be rated above that.

Waters that have been treated with filtration systems or an alkaline water ionizer can be the best approach to ensure the water you're consuming is the best alkaline water available. An alkaline water machine will alter the pH balance of tap water. The filter usually activated carbon, removes impurities and pollutants. Then, through a process of electrolysis, it splits the hydrogen ions and minerals. This process then splits the water into two sections, alkaline and oxidized. The alkaline water can be used for healthy hydration, and the oxidized water can be used for cleaning (fruits, vegetables, kitchen floors, or windows).

Depending on the budget, and your preference, you can purchase either a countertop or under-cabinet model. These models can range from $500-2000. A reverse osmosis system prepares drinking water by passing it through a series of very fine filters. In this system, each filter serves a specific purpose. Each filter is very fine and removes trace minerals, sediment, and contaminants. Some systems even have filters that will put some substances back into the way – substances such as calcium and magnesium. These systems typically cost less than the counter-top or under-cabinet water ionizers. For the budget conscious, an alkaline water pitcher can prepare alkaline water with adequate quality.

Chapter 8:
WHAT IS AN ALKALINE DIET?

"Let there be work, bread, water, and salt for all."
–Nelson Mandela

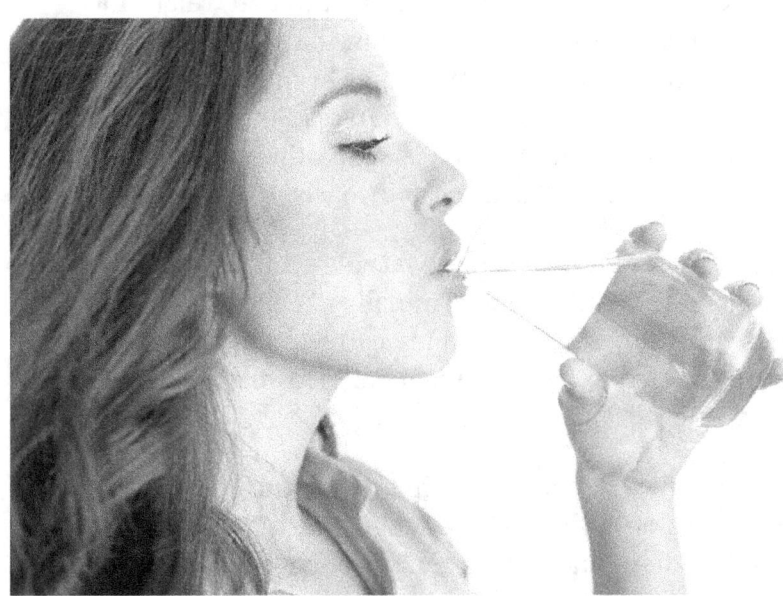

This diet deals not with the alkaline/acid rating of the food itself but the impact the food has on the pH of the body once it has been metabolized. One surprising example is lemon. Although known to be acidic as a citrus, when you add it to water, it then changes the water into alkaline. Similarly, when produce like tomatoes or oranges is eaten, they end up having an alkaline effect on a human body.

The lungs and kidney work diligently to keep the pH of the body closely regulated. A blood rating of 7.4 is typical, and even small variations in that can have big consequences. Part of the appeal of the alkaline diet is not actually reducing or changing the acidity rating of the blood, it is to help the systems that regulate the bodywork less hard. Diets that are alkaline lead to higher levels of magnesium in cells. This mineral is required for a lot of enzyme systems within the human body. It is also necessary for activating vitamin D. These elevated levels may also assist with slowing the aging process and with the preservation of muscle mass.

If what we put in our mouths generally creates a high-acid load – substances such as animal protein, grains, soda, and beer – our systems can get overloaded. If the rest of our diet consists of potassium and minerals, such as fruits and vegetables like spinach, bananas, mushrooms, and wheatgrass, then those high acid loads are processed continuously through the kidneys. Over time, this can damage the kidneys, create kidney stones, and weaken the bones. With too much acid, the storage of minerals to help the system is constantly being depleted to replenish the stores. Guidelines for this diet call for a daily regime of at least 50% plant foods, with at least 25% of those being consumed raw. Since cooking destroys nutrients, raw is best.

The alkaline diet approach originated from theories related to osteoporosis. It has been promoted by alternative health practitioners as a way to reduce the acidity in the body. Without a predominance of acid, then disease cannot develop. This research may have stemmed from the research done by a French biologist by the name of Claude Bernard. During his research,

Bernard was keeping rabbits for his experiments. He changed the diet of his lab rabbits from a primarily herbivore diet to a most carnivore diet. Bernard then tested the urine output of the rabbits and discovered that the more they strayed from their herbivore roots, the more acidic their urine output became. Bernard then made the assumption that we could change our diets to change the body chemistry.

A number of celebrities follow this movement and swear by both the alkaline diet and drinking alkaline water. Most are very vocal about using the diet plan to prepare for upcoming roles. The American public knows that celebrities work very hard to alter body shapes and weight for potential and upcoming movie roles. Most of them have a support staff that researches and investigates the best way for them to meet those goals. Celebrities like Gwyneth Paltrow, Victoria Beckham, Jennifer Aniston, Jared Leto, Kirsten Dunst, and Alicia Silverstone have all expressed their support for this diet at one point or another. But as with other diet trends, preferences and outlooks can change yearly, monthly, even on a daily basis.

One of the biggest advocates of the alkaline diet called Dr. Young faced a criminal trial in 2016 for practicing medicine without a license and for defrauding terminally ill cancer patients. Although Dr. Young holds a doctorate in nutrition, it is from an unaccredited university. The first trial was deadlocked, and the second trial led to five months in jail. However, even with these developments, Dr. Young still advocates his alkaline approach.

In a conflicting view, The American Institute for Cancer Research does not advocate this type of diet in preventing the development of cancer nor in the treatment of cancer. Their position is that body chemistry cannot be influenced by diet; our body systems are finely attuned to keep the chemistry at specific levels, and those levels are controlled specifically by internal body systems.

However, the outline of foods listed in the alkaline diet includes those that one would naturally assume would be beneficial to health – lots of vegetables and fruits, avoiding processed sugars. It seems like a common sense approach to a diet, regardless of what it is called. To increase the alkaline balance of the human body, a wholesome, vegetable-centered diet can be followed as well. Diet should consist of approximately 60-80% alkaline forming foods with only 20-40% made up of acid-forming foods.

Specific foods create too much acid in the system and should be avoided. Also known as the alkaline ash diet, the acid-ash diet, and the pH diet, this type of diet skyrocketed in popularity around 2013 when Victoria Beckham (formerly of the Spice Girls) tweeted about following this approach. Some of its other names came about because the eating plan is based on the consumption of alkaline foods in place of acid foods. When a person eats, their bodies burn the food for fuel. When it's been metabolized for calories, ash is left behind. That ash can either be acidic or alkaline. Advocates claim that the ash left behind can affect how acidic the body is. If the ash is alkaline, it is protective and can be beneficial.

This approach focuses on taking in mostly raw fruits and vegetables. This assists the body in maintaining an alkaline state. If the body doesn't get enough alkaline from the diet, then the body will call on the mineral reserves found in blood, bone, and tissues to balance the system. This can lead to deficiencies of several key minerals.

In the end, once everything's said and done, a perfect balance is what we should all strive for. Drinking alkaline water may help to reduce acid levels in the stomach, but it could also reduce them too much. Those acid levels help to kill bacteria, so in fact, too much alkaline in the system may lead to some gastrointestinal issues and other symptoms, such as:

- Nausea
- Hand tremors
- Vomiting
- Tingling in face/extremities
- Confusion
- Muscle twitching
- Metabolic alkalosis

On the flip-side, a diet low in acid-producing foods might possibly help to prevent kidney stones, improve heart health, keep bones and muscles strong, reduce lower back pain, lower the risk of developing Type 2 diabetes, and reduce muscle wasting. This diet will also assist in helping to balance the sodium to potassium ratio, as potassium is present in a number of raw fruits and vegetables. The ratio of potassium to sodium used to be (and still should be) 10:1. Unfortunately, with modern diets of processed convenience foods, that ratio has dropped to 1:3. People now consume three times more sodium over potassium, and thus, most people suffer from a potassium/magnesium deficiency.

To correct this, the best foods to eat include fruits, vegetables, soybeans, tofu, nuts, seeds, and legumes. The worst foods, or those that should be avoided at all costs, are dairy, eggs, meat, most grains, processed foods, alcohol, caffeine, wheat, milk, peanuts, walnuts, fish, shellfish, high-sodium foods, lunch-meat, processed cereal, pasta, rice, and bread. Under this diet approach, protein intake is generally limited to plant-based sources such as beans, tofu, etc. More best foods are listed below.

Best Foods

- Alfalfa grass
- Almonds (protein)
- Avocado
- Barley grass
- Broccoli
- Cabbage
- Celery
- Citrus
- Cucumber
- Dates
- Endive
- Figs
- Garlic
- Ginger
- Grapefruit

- Green beans
- Jicama
- Kale
- Lima beans (protein)
- Mushrooms
- Navy beans (protein)
- Oregano
- Raisins
- Red Beets
- Ripe bananas
- Spinach
- Tomatoes
- Watermelon
- Wheatgrass

When following the alkaline diet, some supplements and nutritional shakes are also a good idea to boost vitamins and minerals. One of the best, wheatgrass, is a nutrient-rich member of the wheat family. This supplement can be purchased in liquid, tablet, powder, or capsule forms. Frequently, it is added to a morning smoothie. Wheatgrass can add a string of nutrients such as amino acids, calcium, iron, magnesium, chlorophyll, and vitamins A, C, and E. This mixture can help to boost immunity and rid the body of waste. Research is still continuing as to the effectiveness of wheatgrass, so it is difficult to assess the veracity of the claims. Wheatgrass may also cause nausea or constipation, and if you are intolerant to gluten, wheatgrass might not be the best choice for you. Since wheatgrass is processed raw, it is also eaten raw, which means it might possibly be subject to bacteria and mold. As with anything else stated herein, this may be of benefit but should be thoroughly researched before being added to your daily regime.

Supplements can boost the effectiveness of an alkaline diet. But as with any supplement, the dosage and combination are important. These supplements include:

- Potassium citrate: this can help to prevent recurrence of calcium oxalate stones in the kidney. One study showed that potassium citrate/bicarbonate may completely dissolve kidney stones. For the best and most effective combination, potassium citrate (99 mg) and magnesium citrate (300-400 mg) should be taken in combination.
- Calcium: helps to decrease the effects of hypertension, acidosis, and offsets bone demineralization. Calcium, 1000 mg taken daily, should always be balanced with magnesium, and vitamins D3 and K2.
- Vitamin D: also known as the sunshine vitamin, this aids in the absorption of magnesium and calcium.
- Glutamine: something needed in small doses compared to other supplements, glutamine is an amino acid that plays a role in homeostasis. This replicates a substance that is produced by the body to remove excess ammonia.
- Green superfoods: there are a number of these available on the market, including spirulina or chlorella – these are blends that, in powder form, can be added to your morning smoothie. Some are a blend of various types of grasses, such as barley, wheat, or alfalfa. Some other things to look out for in the list of ingredients are artificial sweeteners like xylitol. Others feel that it should be primarily vegetables with very little high sugar fruits; low sugar fruits like grapefruits, lemons, tomatoes, and limes are fine to be on the ingredient list. Some feel that mushrooms should not be on the list either as ingesting fungus it not beneficial for the human body.

As the alkaline diet is now on animal proteins and meat, a daily healthy fat should be added either in the form of omega oils or coconut oil. For the omega, there are ongoing debates on whether omega-3 is sufficient or if a blend of omega 3-6-9 should be followed. The perfect blend of omegas is more important, but while the balance between the three is also crucial, of the three supplements, omega-3 is the one we are more likely to be short in ingesting through natural foods. As an alternative, there are a number of plant-based protein powders that can be added to smoothies to replace the lack that the removal of animal protein in the diet will create. Plants such as peas, hemp, and sprouted brown rice can provide a huge amount of protein hand-in-hand with amino acids.

If you are following the alkaline diet to assist in the reduction of inflammation, there are a number of supplements that are currently hot on the market that might be of interest as well. One of the biggest marketed right now is curcumin. This is a compound under the turmeric family that has strong anti-inflammatory properties. Along with this is turmeric itself, another powerful anti-inflammatory that is popular with those that follow alternative health supplements.

As with any supplement that you put in your body, research should be done to ensure they are of the highest quality. Once you choose which supplements to take, do the research and ensure that the supplements are high quality, organic, non-GMO, has no sugar, fillers, or binding agents.

Some of the critics of the diet, however, cite how little reliable, scientific evidence exists to support this diet. In addition, some acids (fatty acids and amino acids) are essential building blocks to life, so eliminating all acidic foods would be detrimental. The list of foods is very limited as well and requires the elimination of some beneficial proteins like meat, dairy, and eggs. Again, as with the alkaline water, critics argue that external sources cannot change the pH level of bodily fluids and internal systems.

Some great recipes for alkaline smoothies to help boost energy and adjust your alkaline levels are laid out in the next pages.

Alkaline Smoothie

- Almond butter (2-4 oz.)
- Almond milk (16 oz.)
- Banana (1)
- Berries (8 oz.)
- Chia (1 T)
- Fresh spinach (16 oz.)

Blend everything except chia seeds. Stir in the chia by hand.

Grapefruit Smoothie

- Coconut milk (8 oz.)
- Grapefruit (1)
- Fresh spinach (8 oz.)
- Sweetener – a pinch of your preferred

Blend all together.

Green Smoothie

- Banana (half of 1)
- Fresh basil (2 oz.)
- Coconut milk – unsweetened (12 oz.)
- Flaxseed (1 T)
- Kale (8 oz.)
- Strawberries (3 large)

Blend everything together.

Tropical Smoothie

- Coconut water (2 oz.)
- Shredded coconut (2 tsp.)
- Honey (1 T)
- Mango (4 oz.)
- Pineapple (4 oz.)
- Fresh spinach (4 oz.)
- Yogurt (4 oz.)

Blend everything together.

Energizing Smoothie

- Almond milk (4 oz.)
- Avocado (half)
- Broccoli (16 oz.)
- Cucumber (6 oz.)
- Ice
- Limes (2)
- Spinach (24 oz.)
- Tofu (4 oz.)

Blend all ingredients together.

Super Shake

- Avocado (one-half)
- Chia (1 T)
- Coconut oil (1 tsp.)
- Coconut water (4 oz.)
- Cucumber (5 oz.)
- Ginger (.5 oz.)
- Lime (juice of one lime)
- Kale (8 oz.), stems removed
- Fresh mint (4 oz.)
- Fresh parsley (1 T)
- Sweetener (dash of your preferred)

Blend all ingredients together.

Kiwi Smoothie

- Almonds (4-8)
- Bananas (2)
- Blueberries (8 oz.)
- Honey (3 T)
- Kiwi (3)
- Yogurt (8 oz.)

Blend all ingredients.

Matcha Smoothie

- Almond milk (8 oz.)
- Banana (1)
- Honey (1 T)
- Ice
- Matcha powder (1 tsp.)

Blend all ingredients.

Chapter 9:
HOW LONG HAS ALKALINE WATER BEEN AROUND?

"We forget that the water cycle and the life cycle are one."
–Jacques Yves Cousteau

The Bottle

Bottled water has a longer history than most people would expect. In fact, bottled water essentially began in 1621 in the United Kingdom with the Holy Well. The oldest bottling plant in the world goes by the name of Malvern Hills. This location was a precursor of the Schweppes bottled water dynasty.

The bottled water trend in the 1600s served essentially the same purpose as modern-day bottled water. It was used to bottle mineral waters that the public thought would benefit their health. Saratoga Spring bottled mineral water and sold them at Jackson's Spa in Boston in 1767. In fact, in the mid-century, Saratoga Springs was producing about 7 million bottles annually.

The public bought these bottles in great quantities because they believed the mineral springs has therapeutic properties, similar to when bathing in the minerals. The public was so enamored of the health effects of mineral water that in 1809, Joseph Hawkins was issued the first patent for "imitation" mineral water. In addition, the sanitary conditions of those times were so questionable that the public felt that they were possibly safer buying water that was bottled at the source, so there were no risks of infectious diseases.

This all timed perfectly with a drop in the price of the production of glass, thereby making the production of the containers a much more affordable option. That meant the production of the containers would no longer be so cost-prohibitive that the average citizen couldn't afford to buy it. However, the sale of bottled water began to decline in the Americas after water chlorination became more widespread. That is, until 1977 when Perrier re-started the market. From there, the bottled water industry has skyrocketed, and in 2016, it surpassed soda as our favorite beverage. This is partially because of the convenience of having water on hand to go with us on our travels, but it is also because most people are trying to make the healthier choice of life-affirming water instead of empty sugar calories.

Originally, when bottled water was first sold and marketed as a health treatment, the production of glass was finally becoming more affordable and therefore made it available to the masses. Now, our modern technology has developed even cheaper, more lightweight alternatives to the glass. But the latest controversy is how safe these new materials are. A number of chemicals are necessary for the chemical composition of plastic, but a few of those have some critics who question the risks they may pose.

Bisphenol A (BPA) is used to prevent cracking in softer plastics by stabilizing the epoxy resins. In the heat, if the bottled water is shipped in containers that are not air-conditioned or if it sits in your hot car for two days after you have unloaded the other groceries, BPA is known to leach into the water. This then can create what is known as bad estrogen (or "faux" estrogen). When your levels of this bad estrogen are high, it can affect your endocrine system and increase your risk of ovarian, prostate, and breast cancers.

There are also studies that suggest BPA can adversely affect children's brains, possibly causing hyperactivity and aggression, as well as affect fetuses. And although the circumstances of the leaching (exposure to heat) seem too specific to be an every-day occurrence, this chemical can be found in a lot more than bottled water and can accumulate in the human system from both food sources and pollution.

A lot of companies are moving away from plastics containing BPA; however, almost all plastics contain BPS, a chemical which is similar and can still affect your endocrine system. In fact, the World Health Organization has indicated that plastics are an endocrine disruptor and that this is a worldwide problem that needs to be seriously considered and addressed.

The damage done to the endocrine system may also explain some of the body weight and obesity problems that are currently exploding worldwide. Hormones, specifically estrogen, directly influence how fat is stored in the body. Plastic toxins can accumulate over years of use and build up in the liver and kidneys. Unfortunately, this isn't limited to the bottled water that we drink; this includes any other beverages and foods that might be exposed to these chemicals.

Polyethylene terephthalate (PET) is an additive which is strong but lightweight. This is the chemical name for polyester. This helps to keep the bottles clear and light. Almost all of the 2-liter bottles that carry soda in the U.S. are made from PET. Some reports indicate that PET bottles since the plastic is so much softer, are almost impossible to clean. This isn't a problem for new plastic, but once the bottles are recycled, the material can then contain fecal matter, saliva, food residues of the previous consumer, and what it has picked up through the recycling process.

This additive has been around for decades, but most people don't even think about this as an ingredient. The question remains as to whether it is safe for perpetual use with food. Again, this chemical is less stable when exposed to high heat conditions or when exposed to ultraviolet light, both of which can cause this chemical to degrade and leach into the water. This chemical additive has become more prevalent with the bad press that BPA has received. Scientists are now doing research into PET to see if it really is a safer alternative. Some research has shown that this additive also has the potential to interfere with estrogen and other reproductive hormones as well.

Phthalates are used to make plastic flexible. This is more commonly connected to the PVC (polyvinyl chloride) pipes that now run through most homes. However, some studies suggest a link between phthalates and liver cancer and sterility in males.

Although plastic has generally been rated safe for public consumption, as a man-made material, it is still a chemical compound that should be fully researched before exposure. And, as with anything, everything in moderation: no one should saturate their lives with any one substance. So, mix it up, use a glass travel bottle, invest in a stainless steel bottle, or use a glass pitcher with filtered mineral water. Pay attention to recycling codes to ensure you are picking the safest ones. Some scientists feel that certain codes reflect safer plastic materials, including ratings 1, 2, 4, and 5.

- Recycling symbol 1: PET rating – most common for single-use bottled beverages. Easy to recycle, lightweight, and inexpensive to manufacture (and therefore less expensive to the consumer). Lower risk of leaching. Recycling rates still need to increase as they are currently at 20%.
- Recycling symbol 2: HDPE (high-density polyethylene) – used primarily for juice bottles and milk jugs but also for things like spreadable butter tubs or yogurt containers. Low risk of leaching and easy to recycle.
- Recycling symbol 4: LDPE (low-density polyethylene) – used most often in shopping bags and squeezable bottles. Less commonly recycled; you must take these to a drop-off center to recycle. Less likely to be found in food containers.
- Recycling symbol 5: PP (polypropylene) – found in syrup bottles, straws, bottle caps, yogurt containers, ketchup bottles, and some medicine bottles. Part of most larger recycling programs. Has a higher melting point, so they're used for containers that need to safely contain hot liquid.

Recycling programs have become commonplace nowadays, and almost every street corner has recycling stations for glass, paper, and plastic. And yet, only a small percentage of materials are still recycled. In fact, although statistics vary, rates range from 20-30%, which means that the large majority of plastic bottles still end up in landfills. Studies show that those bottles could take 450 years to biodegrade. It is up to every one of us to make sure that our choice for healthy water doesn't lead to a more unhealthy choice for the environment.

One alternative that is healthier than plastic is glass bottles. There have no chemicals that can leach into water, and they are easily cleaned and sanitized. But the drawback is that they are fragile and easily broken. This makes them inconvenient for use during workouts or physical activity. Designers are helping people get around that by introducing silicone sleeves.

A second option is stainless steel bottles. They are not breakable, they are easy to sterilize, are lighter than glass, and keep hot and cold beverages at that temperature longer. A drawback is that given enough cycle runs through a dishwasher, some containers may show wear and tear.

The Science

To look at the history of alkaline water, you must first look at both the history of electrolysis and the concept of healthy water. The process of electrolysis has been used since the mid-1700s, although initially, it was not used on water. It was first used to separate water in the 1800s, and the effects of this processed water on plants and animals were studied. Sometime after World War I, both Japan and Russia sought to learn the effects of alkaline water.

The modern uses of ionization came from Michael Faraday, who invented the magneto and dynamo. Faraday, a pioneer in the field of electrical energy, contributed the technology for electrolysis to separate water molecules. At the time he invented it. However, Faraday didn't realize the implications his invention would have on the health industry.

Research into negative ions and their role first began as early as the 1850s in Russia. Scientists in Russia did most of the preliminary research on ionized water. These scientists noticed that positive ions were detrimental, so the assumption was made that negative ions must indeed be beneficial. They experimented with simple electrolysis where an anode and cathode were put into water at the same time, creating both positive and negative ions. Those ions canceled each other out.

This discovery led to the first development of ionizers in Russia in the early 1900s. Russian scientists, influenced by Faraday's technology, used what they knew to investigate the relationship between water with longevity and health. This research and experimentation may have given rise to the novel Lost Horizons by James Hilton. That novel led to the film about the search for a hidden paradise by the name of Shangri-La. That land, hidden away from the world, was blessed with eternal life and health. The parallel is then drawn between alkaline water and the fountain of youth.

Because of the radiation fall-out from the Cold War, Russia was compelled to continue and expand their research into the benefits of alkaline water and negative ions. In fact, alkaline water is shown to help people who are undergoing radiation/chemotherapy treatments.

In the 1950s, Japan had begun joining in the experiments, conducting most of them on plants and animals as they tried to find the effect of negative ions on living materials. The Japanese agricultural universities focused their research on functional water technology. In fact, the acidic water, which is the second part or byproduct of the process, is actually used today by nurseries in order to preserve flowers longer.

The first ionizer was then made and sold in 1958. Initially, the ionization units were huge and were mainly used in hospitals as a supplemental treatment for patients. Then, in 1960, an agricultural/medical research institute was founded with the primary directive of looking into the wide-spread health benefits of ionized water. By 1966, the Japanese Health Ministry had officially approved the ionizer as a "health-improving medical device." Korea followed suit and approved similar uses a decade later. Water ionizers are now pretty standard in Japanese culture with over 30 million citizens now having access to ionized water (either through a home unit or public units).

~

The field of research on alkaline water was primarily about the trends found based on the health and longevity of various regions of the world: Hunza in the Himalayas, the Andes Mountains, Shin-Chan in China, and the Caucasus in Azerbaijan. In those regions, although diets and lifestyles were different, the properties of their water were similar to each other but different from the rest of the world. And in those regions, people were healthier and lived longer. Scientists began looking at the structure of the water, and they noticed some fundamental differences.

As mentioned earlier, the Hunza Valley in the Himalayas is a prime example of a blue zone. Dr. Henri Coanda was a Romanian scientist instrumental in fluid dynamics; he won a Nobel Prize and held over 600 patents. He developed an interest in the lifespan of certain regions around the globe; the regions that were called "blue zones" are areas whose populace seemed to have longer, healthier lives. Dr. Coanda made an arduous trek to the region in the Himalayas to see if he could find out why.

The Hunza Valley, only 100 miles long and the subject of a few groups of explorers, scraped out a living by raising goats on the side of the mountain and barely raised enough crops to feed themselves and their families. The soil quality was so poor that both animal and the human fecal matter was put directly into the crops to help with fertilization. But the very source of life seemed to be the aqueduct that fed water to the village. Dr. Coanda found the water properties of Hunza were different. There is a longevity in the area that well exceeds the normal standards. In addition, the literacy rate is also above 95%, again well above the normal standards. Dr. Coanda, "the father of fluid dynamics," spent about 60 years studying the Hunza water, and when he retired Dr. Patrick Flanagan took over the research.

Flanagan had been recognized as one of the most promising scientists at that time. Flanagan began his investigation in the five regions identified with long-lived inhabitants. As Flanagan began studying the different regions, he found the the diet and habits of the people were all different, but the similarities in the water sources in all regions caught his eyes.

At first, it was thought that the fact that the source of the water was a glacier was most important. Coming from a glacier meant that the water was filled to the brim with natural minerals, silica, and electrolytes. However, after some more in-depth research, Flanagan found that the surface tension of the water was lower than typical water. Typical water is at a rating of 73, and Hunza waterfalls at 67. This type of water was then nicknamed "glacial milk" and "Hunza water."

Flanagan was so impressed by the quality and effectiveness of the water that he began a search to create his own version of the beneficial water. Flanagan created a 33-step process using nano-colloidal silicates to come up with a product by the name of Microclusters which can absorb 300% more than a comparable mineral without the boost. As his research continued, Flanagan found that the glacier water also exhibited another trait, an extra hydrogen electron. This extra, negatively-charged hydrogen ion was the perfect catalyst to act as an antioxidant.

Once again, research continued to find another piece of the puzzle regarding the effectiveness of water from the region. Another factor was that the mineral make-up was a new type of mineral colloid that was smaller than most trace minerals. The colloid minerals were so small that almost 2.5 million would fit on the head of a pin, and this makes them readily absorbable by the human body. This nanotechnology took water technology to the next level.

The water from Hunza comes from melted glaciers, contained certain silicate minerals, and has some very specialized properties:

1. It contains negatively-charged hydrogen ions which are powerful antioxidants. This neutralizes free radicals in the body.
2. It closely resembles, structurally, the water found in the cells of the human body.
3. It can move between the cells of the body, helping to flush out the toxins, and it more readily absorbs into the cells.
4. It is highly alkaline – which means that it may help to neutralize acids in the body. The thought is that cancer and disease cannot exist in an alkaline state, so if the body is more alkaline than acid, then there'll be no disease.
5. It contains silica which, in general, helps to chelate heavy metals out of the body, pulling mercury, lead, cadmium, and aluminum out.

The alkaline state of the water was a later discovery. As hydrogen is the fuel of life, any water that is high in hydrogen would be more beneficial. The food we consume releases hydrogen, which is then burned by oxygen, which then releases energy – the fuel that runs our very bodies. This burning fuel mixture is a three-part mixture: hydrogen, carbohydrates, and oxygen. Hydrogen is the energy source and makes up about 90% of the mass of the entire universe. Is it just a coincidence that water with a predominance of hydrogen would be anything less than life-giving to the human body?

Some Takeaways

Every enzyme reaction in the human body uses negative ionized hydrogen with a free electron. We get these negative ionized hydrogen from foods we eat, water we drink, and supplements we take. The best way to get them is to only eat pure, raw, organic food and drink lots of fresh organic juices – but in the typical diet and lifestyle, most people don't accomplish that and need as much help as possible.

One simple way to reduce acid in the system and to raise your alkaline levels can be something as free as deep breathing exercises. When we do deep breathing, we increase our oxygen intake which helps to relieve stress, cleanse the body of toxins, and improve digestion. When we breathe rapidly and shallowly, we stimulate the nervous system, activating our stress responses. Especially shallow breathing can create an imbalance and allow an excess of carbon dioxide in the blood. This excess can lead to an overly acidic state.

Deep, diaphragmatic breathing is one of the first steps to overall health. Deep breaths increase oxygen in the system, cleaning the body on a cellular level, improving digestion, and relieving stress hormones. It should be deep, even breathing – deep breaths, filling the lower part of your lungs – your diaphragm – inhale, wait for four counts, and exhale for four counts. Do this every morning and every evening for several minutes.

In addition to breathing, sleep is very important as well. The basic building block of health helps maximize the digestion, mental clarity, blood sugar levels, and hormone balance. Hormonal imbalance is one of the top reasons for our cravings of refined sugar and carbohydrates, which leads to a more acidic diet. Everyone who has kept at it until late in the night working or preparing for a test knows that at 3:00 in the morning, when you just can't stand another five minutes of Shakespeare, a chocolate bar, a cup of coffee, or soda with loads of caffeine could help revive us. Unfortunately, such cravings are bad for our health. In addition, when you are short on sleep, your adrenal and thyroid glands kick up their secretion of stress hormones which creates an acidic condition. This may lead to inhibit the digestive system.

Exercise is also great for reducing acidity in the body. Movement, even exercise as basic as taking a walk, can help boost our internal balance and move waste products through the body so it can more easily eliminate them. Although aerobic exercise is the best, any exercise can help reduce the accumulation of acid in the system. A walk is not as aerobic, but a simple walk in a serene location will also help lower the stress hormones in the body. Specifically, exercise lowers the levels of adrenaline and cortisol and stimulates the production of endorphins.

Chapter 10:
HOW DO YOU TEST IF WATER IS ALKALINE?

"Water is fluid, soft, and yielding. But water will wear away rock, which is rigid and cannot yield. As a rule, whatever is fluid, soft, and yielding will overcome whatever is rigid and hard. This is another paradox; what is soft is strong."
–Lao Tzu

There are a number of different ways you can test the pH levels of water. Some are as simple as the science experiments that you used to perform in science class. On the market, there are now portable, small electronic pH meters that you can use to test your water. Each of those comes with a set of instructions that should be explicitly followed to ensure the results are accurate.

You can also use pH test strips. These should not be confused with common litmus paper as they differ in usage (litmus paper simply identifies an acid or base solution, but does not give an accurate rating). The pH strip, once exposed to the liquid solution, will change color. The strength of the acids/bases on each bar changes the color of the strip and will correspond to the color chart kit that comes with the testing kit. The pH scale, the number that matches the color chart, rates the level of acidity/alkalinity of the water.

The pH scale runs from 0 to 14 (although substances can actually fall outside that range). Neutral substances rate close to a 7; acidic are below, and alkaline is above. The pH scale is a logarithmic scale, which means that the differences of a single integer actually represent a difference of ten times; i.e., a pH of 2 is actually ten times more acidic than a substance with a rating of 3 and 100 times more acidic than a substance with a pH of 4. This sliding scale also functions the same way for alkaline substances; the difference in one integer will mean a tenfold difference in alkalinity.

Although the test kits come with instructions which should be explicitly followed, the typical procedures usually go thus:

1. Collect the water in a small, clean, sanitized container. Make sure the electronic probe is clean if you are using that form. Remove the pH strips from the kit if you are using that form.
2. If you are using an electronic probe, you may have to calibrate it according to the manufacturer's specifications.
3. If you are using an electronic probe, you will need to know the temperature of the water and to input the temperature into the sensor so that measurements will be accurate.
4. For the electronic probe, insert the tip into the water. Wait the specified time as per the instructions.

5. If you are using the pH strips, put the paper in water. Wait until the paper registers and compare to the color chart that is provided with the kit.

Chapter 11:
HOW ESSENTIAL IS ALKALINE WATER?

"Water is the lifeblood of our bodies, our economy, our nation, and our wellbeing."
–Stephen Johnson

A human body can go more than three weeks without food, but 60% of the body needs water to function. This means that death from lack of water may happen in less than a week. Water is essential to the hydration of the human body. Dehydration can greatly affect how you feel, and losing even as little as 2% of the body's water content can change your entire state. Worse, a fluid loss of 1.59% is detrimental to the brain, affecting memory and raising levels of anxiety and fatigue. Hydration leads to more energy. It can prevent headaches, relieve constipation, improve focus, reduce oxidative stress, improve moods, prevent hangovers, and possibly prevent any recurrence of kidney stones. The U.S. Federal Emergency Management Agency (FEMA) recommends storing one (1) gallon of water per person per day for a three (3) day supply in case of an emergency. We simply can't live without it.

Water is an amazing substance. It can take many forms – solid, liquid, and gas – and each of those forms have some type of benefit. Water in the form of glaciers can change the very landscape. Water in the form of vapor is one of the substances that help to warm the very atmosphere we live in. In liquid form, when we ingest the right kinds of water, it can nourish our bodies.

If we drink the right kinds of water, we can take the process from a simple act of hydration to a boost to our very health. The health benefits of alkaline water carrying all of the right minerals and trace elements elevate a sip of water to something more – an essential building block of life.

Claims by the supporters of alkaline water promise it will help to detoxify the body and combat the negative effects of a diet high in acid. In fact, some people suffering from osteoporosis and abnormal renal acidification undergo alkali therapy. This consists of taking ammonium chloride on a daily basis. This type of treatment isn't possible just with drinking alkaline water, but it certainly is one step in the entire process. Testing has also shown that drinking water with a pH of at least 8.8 inactivates human pepsin, a substance that contributes to acid reflux. Ingesting normal tap water with a pH lower than 7 didn't have any effect on acid reflux.

If we add more hydrogen into the mix, those benefits can change on a large scale. In addition to the capabilities listed in the first chapter, drinking alkaline water can counteract the external/internal factors that may raise the acidity of the body. Factors that might raise acid levels are:

- Alcohol use
- Antibiotics use
- Artificial sweeteners
- Caffeine intake
- Chronic stress
- Drug use
- Excessive amounts of exercise
- Excessive animal/meat protein
- Excessive hormones from food, beauty products, or plastic
- Exposure to chemicals or radiation (such as cell phones or microwave use)
- Food coloring and preservatives in our food
- Little/no exercise
- Low levels of fiber
- Low nutrient-rich diet
- Pesticides and herbicides
- Pollution

Although any doctor will tell you that hydration is important and your research leads you to choose alkaline water to help to balance the system, it doesn't change the fact that you still have other choices to make. You don't want to undo the benefits of that alkaline water by choosing a source that is not optimum. For instance, do not choose dead water just for the one benefit of ingesting alkaline. In addition, the water should also hold some of the most essential vitamins. Ensure that both sides of this life-giving substance are as beneficial as possible: the alkaline rating of the water should match the mineral content.

There are a number of minerals in healthy water, known as electrolytes, that are essential to the very functioning of our bodies:

Sodium

- Helps to keep fluids in balance
- Controls nerve function
- Regulates muscle function

When there is too little, effects include brain dysfunction, sluggishness, confusion, muscle twitches, and seizures.

Potassium

- Basis of cells

- Involved in nerve function
- Supports muscle function

When there is too little, effects include abnormal heart rhythm, vomiting, diarrhea, weakness, cramps.

Calcium

- Formation of bones and teeth
- Muscle contraction
- Blood clotting
- Normal heart rhythm

When there is too little, the system starts siphoning calcium out of the bones and produces an excess amount of parathyroid hormones.

Magnesium

- Formation of bones and teeth
- Nerve function
- Muscle function
- This enzyme is used by a lot of other bodily functions
- Tied to metabolism of calcium and potassium

When there is too little, you can experience nausea, vomiting, sleepiness, weakness, muscle spasm, tremors, and loss of appetite.

Phosphate

- Formation of bones and teeth
- Building block of cell energy
- Building block of cell membranes
- Building block of DNA

When there is too little, you can experience muscle weakness, stupor, coma, death, weak bones, and loss of appetite.

There was a period of time wherein many advocate pure drinking water. The more purified and the more processed, the better. The school of thought was that removing all of the bad contaminants was worth the loss of the good minerals. Once this trend began, some very tuned-in doctors noticed that people who consumed a lot of this purified water were experiencing a whole other set of symptoms. For example, people who switched over to consuming only reverse osmosis water suffered from an extreme loss of bone density. The instances of bone density loss can be linked directly to the dead water. In fact, those same critics indicate that there is a connection between over-consuming alkaline water and the over-alkalization of the digestive system and a compromised immune function. These same critics compare alkaline ionized water to hybrid fruits and vegetables, commonly referred to as GMOs (genetically modified organisms).

One side benefit of alkaline water that isn't readily apparent but that is still a big perk is the process of electrolysis itself. When using a water ionizer, as the water separates alkaline water and acid water are both created. Alkaline water is beneficial to our bodies, but the acid water can serve as a host of possible good uses. These would include:

- Household cleaning: acidic water is better suited to cleaning kitchen counters, the handle of the refrigerator, the very surfaces that your family touches every day. Since this highly acidic water is good at killing bacteria, it is exceptionally efficient at disinfecting surfaces. In addition, to use this water on dishcloths and sponges will diminish odors and slow bacteria growth.
- Food cleaning: using acidic water to clean fruits, vegetables, and meats can help to prevent contamination.
- First aid: acidic water is good for cleaning cuts and minor burns as it kills bacteria. It can even help with the pain and inflammation caused by minor burns.
- Beauty: helps to treat acne, skin spots, and other skin conditions. Using acidic water to wash your face and remove makeup can help. In the shower, rinsing your hair with acid water before shampooing will help to prevent hair loss, dandruff, or itchy scalp. To use acid water to shave helps to protect against shaving rash. Highly beneficial is to add 1.5-3 gallons of acid water to a bath. In addition, if you can, use organic and natural brand that are made with the safest of ingredients. However, there is a benefit to using the alkaline water for bathing as well. There are some trains of thought that believe an alkaline bath at a pH level of 8.5 most closely simulates amniotic fluid. There are several products on the market that can help to recreate the chemical balance of that amniotic fluid, assisting to flush toxins from the body. These bath soaks include a mixture of sea salts, minerals, baking soda, and various gemstones. In fact, the soles of the feet are a very good location for pulling toxins out of the body. Doing a detox foot bath several times a week for six (6) months will gently remove toxins from the body. Too much or too long of a soak removes the toxins too quickly and may cause some discomfort. Be careful not to buy dead sea salt as an ingredient as they are actually more acidic and may defeat the purpose.
- Medicinal: soaking afflicted feet for 20-30 minutes in acidic water can help alleviate athletes foot; soaking afflicted hands for 20-30 minutes helps to treat nail fungus. It can also help with insect bites and chapped hands.
- Miscellaneous: acid water is especially good in the kitchen to help eliminate strong odors on your hands – e.g., the odors of onions and garlic. A little acid water mixed with your favorite essential oils can make garlic odors disappear. In addition, if you're lucky enough to receive some fresh flowers, putting them in a vase of acid water will help to keep the flowers fresher for longer. In fact, watering all of your houseplants with acid water will make them green and healthy.

Closing Thoughts

As with anything else in life, choosing our drinking water also comes down to common sense. As there is not magic fountain of youth, no pill you can take that can suddenly roll back two decades of life, using common sense is the best approach left to us. For example, as everyone knows, water is beneficial. But in researching the topic and finding out that dead water, which is lacking in natural minerals that the body can use for healthful benefits, may indeed actually be leaching minerals out of the body, then that type of water should not be the type of hydration you would want to seek out.

While some practitioners feel that you can raise the levels of alkalinity by ingesting alkaline water, other feel that too much alkaline water may affect the natural balance sustained by the body. In this case, possibility drinking nothing but alkaline water might not be the best approach either. A number of water sommeliers have indicated that there are different flavors and different mouth-feels for different types of water – and each type of water can accompany a different meal or purpose. Therefore, a delicate balance should once again be established by interspersing alkaline water with tap water, distilled water, purified water, or other preference.

CITATIONS:

www.healthline.com

www.precisionnutrition.com

www.santevia.com

www.mnn.com – Mother Nature Network

www.water-for-health.co.uk

www.prestiguewater.com

www.ncbi.nlm.nih.gov (U.S. National Library of Medicine – NIH)

www.alkalinewatermachinereviews.com

https://draxe.com

www.bottledwater.org (International Bottled Water Association)

https://bodyecology.com

Drinking Water Research Foundation – Bottled Water and Tap Water Just the Facts, October 2011

www.merckmanuals.com

:

Wheatgrass

The Guidebook for Enjoying a World of Health Benefits of a Superfood

Table of Contents

Introduction

I am so glad you took time out of your busy schedule to download your copy of *Wheatgrass: The Guidebook for Enjoying a World of Health Benefits of a Superfood.* Thank you. The following chapters will discuss some of the many different ways wheatgrass can provide you with essential vitamins and minerals. It is also rich in protein containing 17 amino acids, which are the building blocks of protein.

The young grass is of the wheat plant called Triticum aestivum. By the way, it is also gluten-free and can be milled down into a fine powder that is used to prepare juices (which are also called "shots"), smoothies, and salads. It comes in the form of powders, capsules, tablets, and pills.

Wheatgrass is very versatile, and it's not new. Many professional athletes have used it to remain healthy. The American diet is packed with fats. If you find yourself pushing the greens to the side and eat fast food on a regular basis, you may need to consider adding wheatgrass to your diet plan.

Don't worry, this isn't a gimmick, and it isn't that expensive. You can learn how to grow your own if you like to play in the dirt. There are plenty of books offered on this subject in today's market, so thanks again for choosing this one! Every effort was made to ensure that it is full of as much useful information as possible. Please enjoy!

Let's begin!

Chapter 1: Wheatgrass—Nutrition & Expense

Wheatgrass is a member of the wheat family and is derived from the red wheat berry. The grain produced is high in vitamins, enzymes, chlorophyll, vital amino acids, and antioxidants. During the growing process, the plant is green and begins to develop a shaft that produces the small grains on the top that can be harvested. The grass stage at about seven days produces growth of 6–9 inches. It is cut at this point before the grains are produced and dried to use as a powder.

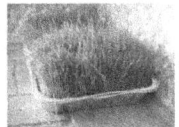

Nutrition

The Superfood is a source of dietary fiber, potassium, Vitamin A, Vitamin C, Vitamin K, Vitamin E (alpha-tocopherol), zinc, selenium, copper, and magnesium. Its source of protein is less than 28 grams. One shot of wheatgrass juice will supply 10% of your daily iron and about 6% of the Vitamin C needed daily.

The addition of "complementary" amino acids to the wheatgrass may yield a much more complete source of protein. It can also improve the quality of many of the restrictive diets. The nutrient content of wheatgrass juice is roughly estimated to be equivalent to dark leafy veggies.

There is a bit of speculation through the popular belief that the B12 is not contained in the superfood wheatgrass plant. It is the byproduct of the living microorganisms that live on the plants or in the existing soil. Therefore, according to the USDA National Nutrient Database, the superfood does not contain the B12 vitamin.

Consider Protein

You need to know what form of wheatgrass you will be consuming before you know the protein content. One shot of wheatgrass equals about one gram of protein. That is not much considering the 46 grams women need daily. Men need 56 grams. There are an additional 2 grams of protein per each 8-gram scoop.

You need the protein to repair your tissues, cells, and muscles. According to the Harvard School of Public Health, the amino acids in protein-rich foods also aid in the production of new proteins.

The Cost

You can purchase a pouch of wheatgrass for about $11.00 USD. That is 30 servings or a 1-month supply.

Consider this simple drink of water. Mix one teaspoon of wheatgrass (flavor of your choosing) to one glass of water with a squeeze of lemon. Make it even healthier by using filtered or mineral water. The freshness of the superfood is invigorating and gets you off to the right start for a minimal cost.

Now, let us see how healthy the superfood is as part of your diet regimen!

Chapter 2: Health Benefits

Are you seeking a way to raise your energy levels or trying to overcome various ailments? You can drastically improve your body's natural ability to manage stress and heal itself by boosting the quality of the foods you eat. Wheatgrass can provide you with a great deal that nutrition.

The Components of Wheatgrass

Your overall health and well-being depend on what you consume. The Mayo Clinic notes that you will receive nutrition packed in each serving including:

Antioxidants

Your body is cleansed and toxins are removed when the wheatgrass is consumed. The nutrients comb across a buildup of plaque and push it off to clear the arteries. It can also benefit you by:

- Fighting off cancer
- Improving arthritis
- Removing cataracts
- Reducing premature aging
- Avoiding or repairing damage to the arteries

The antioxidants will strive to improve your health and remove the toxins stored throughout your body that is causing the disease and inflammation. Studies conducted in 2006 indicated a higher antioxidant level with wheatgrass versus other vegetables.

Chlorophyll

Chlorophyll is a protein found in plant composition that is similar to human red blood cells. It is beneficial if you have gastrointestinal issues. It flushes the colon and helps release disease triggers and improves your digestion.

Your body can help use heavy minerals including calcium as it should be by entering the bloodstream faster than many other foods. It assimilates calcium and other beneficial nutrients so that your tissues can rebuild at a faster rate.

If you have issues with bad breath, wheatgrass can help deodorize that as well.

You can better ward off infections because of its antioxidants assist and help fight any inflammation as it attacks your body.

Wheatgrass works as a detoxing agent to remove portions or all of the toxins that cause cancer. Carcinogen substances are eliminated when you consume chlorophyll. Chlorophyllin is a derivative of this substance.

The production of hemoglobin and red blood cells are also promoted by wheatgrass. Hemoglobin composition is about 75% of the content of your blood. Its iron-rich substances are critical to transport oxygen throughout your cells, body tissues, and organs. The final result is that you are receiving increased energy.

Vitamins A, B, E, C, & K

Some of these vitamins are also antioxidants and are extremely important to your diet plan:

Vitamin A is one of the most important vitamins, and the "superfood" provides twice that amount. Your eyesight is maintained, and you can have healthier skin and can ward off infections and some diseases.

Vitamin C maintains a high count as well with fruits such as oranges, lemons, and kiwis. The superfood has more than one serving of oranges. You develop a stronger immune system and can help fight asthma and allergy symptoms. At the same time, it works as prevention of cardiovascular disease.

B1, B2, B3, B5, By, B12, and B8 are contained in the wheatgrass cabinet. The B vitamins are a great energy source and also prevent cancer and heart disease. Your muscle tone, metabolism, and the maintenance of healthy hair and skin are also evident.

Vitamin K can also help in the prevention of cancer risks, managing clot formation, minimizing menstrual pain, and prevention of the onset/worsening of osteoporosis.

Amino Acids

These organic compounds are a building block related to proteins. These essential vitamins must be consumed in the form of food. Some of these include tryptophan, lysine, isoleucine, and threonine. As an example: Wheatgrass the Superfood has 31 milligrams; you need 20 milligrams in your diet. Leucine should remain around 39 milligrams; the superfood provides you with 57 milligrams.

You will also receive many other benefits including iron, magnesium, and calcium. The benefits overweigh many of the possible side effects. However, each person is different and may have different reactions to the superfood.

Let's discover some of those issues.

Chapter 3: Risks—Side Effects & Precautions

You know all of the benefits of using wheatgrass, but what about the possible side effects? Just like any other product, not everyone receives the same benefits and some may suffer from side effects. It is possible that, since it is grown in the soil and consumed raw, a risk of contamination does exist. The long-term usage of wheatgrass— the superfood—is unknown at this time. If you have any side effects, it is best to visit a doctor to discover what the underlying issue may be.

Side Effects

These are some of the issues to consider:

Nausea: It has been reported that wheatgrass juice could cause nausea. It is a sign that you may not tolerate the juice. Some believe it could be in relation with detoxification, but there is no evidence to support this issue. Gluten is a product of wheatgrass, and therefore, individuals who cannot tolerate gluten can endure the aggravated symptoms.

Low-Grade Fever: Once again, a fever is associated with the detoxification process. Your body is expelling toxins. Therefore, the nasal congestion, cough, and mild fever are symptoms of that process. However, if the symptoms don't go away, it's time to visit your doctor to discover the cause.

Headache: As with nausea, your body may not tolerate the juice, and results in a headache. If this occurs, try drinking less and mix with other juices to mask the taste.

Constipation: Some patients discovered the juice cause bouts of constipation. Once again, you should consult your physician because it could be a sign of an underlying cause other than the wheatgrass.

Allergies: If you consume wheatgrass in the juice or pill form, you could develop allergies because of the overproduction of specific chemicals within the superfood. You may suffer from circulatory issues that can cause the above issues including cramping, nausea, diarrhea, and vomiting. You may also suffer from congestion or shortness of breath. Another possibility is a rash after drinking the juice.

If you cannot tolerate wheat, you need to eliminate wheatgrass from your diet as well. If you suffer from celiac disease, be sure to consult your doctor before using the superfood.

Fatigue & Dizziness: Instead of having large amounts of the superfood juice, try adding a small shot of juice to fresh veggies. Enjoy some of the foods discussed in later chapters.

Loss of Appetite: If you are trying to lose weight, losing the pounds is great, but it may not be as healthy as time passes. There is no scientific evidence to prove it is harmful but has been shown through individual reports.

Stained Teeth: The juices from wheatgrass tend to stain your teeth. Be sure to brush thoroughly after you have your glass of juice to help remedy the situation.

Special Note Concerning Gluten Intolerance

In most cases, wheatgrass is gluten-free because it is made from the stem and leaves. Gluten is found in the kernel of the seed. That is why you must be careful when harvesting to remove the seeds to ensure the gluten does not enter the superfood. If you purchase wheatgrass, be sure it is marked as gluten-free if you have any doubts concerning allergies.

Mold Development

The superfood is grown under moist conditions, and improper plant care can cause mold to develop. During the growing and harvesting process, if you spot mold on the grass, throw the entire section away. You *can* wash it off, but it is best not to take the risk of contamination. Don't second guess it, even though you did take a lot of time to get the plants to this stage. It is not worth it!

The most common type of mold is "blue fuzz" mold, and it is *not* harmful. But just remember, the brown and white types must be disposed of immediately to prevent contamination to the remainder of the crop.

How do you know if the harvest leaves are healthy? One way is to taste the juice. If it is bitter or has a musty aroma, it has mold in it.

Precautions

Before you begin you need to consider these elements:

- If you purchase a wheatgrass powder supplement, the manufacturers advise to store it in the original container. Also, be sure it remains in a dry space.

- Remember the juice is usually in a concentrated form. Taking in less quantity of the juice and adding it to other vegetable juices, and foods will help cover up its taste.

- Always sterilize the growing trays to help prevent contamination.

- If the wheatgrass juice is bitter, it's probably mold. Discard the juice and remove the plant it was taken from.

- If any side effects are bothersome, stop consuming the wheatgrass and contact a doctor.

This segment provided you with the worst-case scenarios. The elements discussed are by no means meant to scare you, but to make you aware of the proper usage of wheatgrass—the superfood.

Chapter 4: Supplies Needed for Growing & Juicing Wheatgrass

As with any healthy food product, you can go to the supermarket or a health food store, but you will know for sure how many nutrients are in your product if it is produced at your location. The superfood doesn't require a lot of space.

The Right Location

A growing tray is the best option, but you can use flowerpots or other containers. You can use them for indoor growing or sprouting so that they can be transplanted outdoors later. Keep these pointers in mind when you begin the process:

1. You will need at least a few inches of soil but easily moved if you need to at some point in time.

2. Use smaller pots and place them around your space if you are in a place without a lot of extra room.

3. Be sure the drainage holes are present in the bottom so that the seeds can grow and not be drowned by sitting water.

4. *Take the Measurements:*

    - For 10 oz. of the juice, you will need ½ lb. of the seed/approximately 1 cup. You will need a smaller tray (10 x 10 is good).

    - For 2 cups of the juice/20 oz., you'll need 1 lb. or 2 cups of the seed. A 17 x 17 tray should be okay.

Start small and experiment to decide how much product you need to grow at a time.

Products & Soil

You will want to get the nutrients from the soil, and it's best to use only organic soils that are nutrient-rich. It doesn't need to be expensive, but you want to be sure it is free of any toxins or chemicals. Wheatgrass is hardy and can be grown in potting mixtures, topsoil, and others. If you prepare an organic compost, be sure its acid levels aren't too harsh, especially for the seeds. It is also important not to purchase nongenetically modified products that possibly pose a risk.

Other Items Needed

There are numerous suppliers to purchase the right wheatgrass seeds. It is always best to research the company before you make your order. The plant has many variations. You will want to search for winter wheat seeds that are harvested to provide a better quality of seed.

You will need a juicer, some time, and a bit of sunlight. It is best to be in an open area to assist during the start of the growing process. Then, you will need to relocate them out of direct sunlight.

Most of your supplies are reusable, and it is best to grow in batches. Start one about a week or so apart from the next group. You will always have a fresh supply of this superfood at hand. The crop rotation also allows for issues such as mold.

Chapter 5: How to Grow Wheatgrass & Juicing

Now, you have the general blueprint for your process.

Guide for Growing—Step-By-Step

The seeds should be readily available before you begin the simple steps.

The Supplies for a 10-x-10 Tray:

- 1 cup wheat sprouting seeds
- 1 jar/bowl for soaking
- Soil enriched with compost, fertilizer/Azomite—if needed
- 10-x-10 growing tray with holes for drainage
    - Growing tray from a garden supply store
    - Plastic deli tray, thoroughly washed
    - Decorative planter, for the growth of ornamental grass
- Plastic lid with air holes—Extra tray to use as a cover

Measure the Wheat Seeds: (Chapter 4)

The Process for Wheat Sprouting:

1. Rinse a ½ cup of the wheat berries and remove any foreign stones or debris.
2. Toss the berries into a 1-quart-size sprouting jar or similar container.
3. Fill with water, then cover with a mesh sprouting screen. Soak overnight or for a minimum of 6 hours.
4. Drain the water from the berries and invert the jar over a bowl (at an angle) so that the berries will continue to drain, but air will circulate.
5. After 8 to 12 hours of draining, rinse and drain once again. Continue the process for 2-3 days.
6. Tiny sprouts will begin to form around this time.
7. Drain well and store or use. The sprouts will keep in a covered container for up to three days in the refrigerator.

How to Use the Berries After Sprouting:

1. Use the berries in soups, bread, salads, and many other recipes (in later chapters). Ferment the berries to make Rejuvelac.
2. Transfer to the soil to grow wheatgrass.
3. Dehydrate and grind into flour for baking.
4. Make sprouted porridge or breakfast cereal.

Growing Wheatgrass:

1. You now see how to sprout the berries. You will notice the sprouts and add ½-1 inch of soil to the growing tray. Gently water to moisten the soil. Don't overwater (avoid puddles).
2. Sprinkle the seeds across the soil and cover.
3. Place the tray in temperatures of 60–80°F using indirect lighting.
4. Cover with a plastic lid (air holes). The grass will grow 1-2 inches, so be sure you allow enough space.
5. Water daily using a sprayer until the seeds root and the grass starts growing.
6. Once the grass reaches 1–2 inches, remove the cover (day 4 approximately).
7. Continue the daily watering.

Harvesting Wheatgrass for Juicing:

1. You will want the grass to be 4–6 inches tall before you harvest. The younger grass is more flavorful than taller grass.
2. Cut just above the roots using a pair of scissors and juice immediately.
3. You can harvest the crop twice, but the nutritional content lowers after the first cutting.
4. Rinse the wheatgrass with cool water and dry with a towel.
5. Wrap it in a dry paper towel and store it in a sealed Ziploc-type baggie until you are ready to use it. It will remain fresh for 1-2 weeks. The temperature in the fridge should be 38°F.

Juicing—Hand in Hand

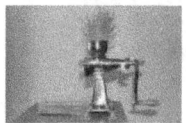

This part if the process begins by using a specialized blender that is fitted as a juicer. You have to break down the cell walls of the plant to remove the nutrients. By juicing, you get all of the nutrition and much faster than if you tried to consume the superfood "as is."

The reason it is best to use a special juicer is that a regular blender or food processor spins rapidly and will oxidize the chlorophyll, thus losing the nutrient. You can use a mortar and pestle for a basic method, but it will take a lot of action to get enough juice to use.

Several manufacturing companies offer a special machine for juicing that are good for extracting the juice from most leafy greens. It is advised by the professionals to use one juicer for wheatgrass—nothing else.

You can purchase a juicer that has a multifunction, whereas one side is for fruits and veggies with the second unit used for your wheatgrass. It depends on how much you want to utilize the equipment. The manual juicer for wheatgrass is the most common. Be sure to consider these elements:

- The unit should be easily cleaned.
- Purchase a juicer that has a base or suction clamp. This will hold the juicer in position as you work the juicer crank.
- Look for one that is easily stored and compact.
- The juicer should have a stainless-steel grinding plate to ensure it will be efficient and easily maintained.
- Most units will have at least a 1-year warranty.
- Most juicers have basic features and accessories. It will need to have a plunger to push the superfood through the opening to prevent injury.
- The unit should be made with toxic polycarbonate products.

Juicers With a Motor

If you don't have the arm strength or time to use the manual juicer, consider these elements of things to look for in a motorized unit:

- It's important the unit is lightweight. Some may be more difficult to handle because of the weight factor.

- Be sure you have a juicer that has a large enough chute that should be 1 ½ inches at a minimum.

- Purchase one with a screen and auger for use.

- The unit should operate with 220 watts of power. That will provide the best possible juice.

- The juicer should have a minimum warranty of 1 year.

Do your research and compare each model. Don't go by the price tag alone.

The Process

Once the wheatgrass has been harvested, cut the superfood in half to make it easier to handle. Add some to the juicer and proceed. You will need to add some water to create a paste.

That's it! Mix the liquid with whatever recipe you choose.

How to Store the Superfood

With the use of an airtight container, you can store your wheatgrass juice in the fridge for 24 to 48 hours. You can use a pitcher to make the pouring easier. Be sure to keep the lid closed to eliminate picking up refrigerator odors.

Are you ready to begin?

Chapter 6: Quality Foods Using Wheatgrass

Adding wheatgrass to your diet is simply accomplished by preparing delicious and healthy foods in your kitchen. The recipes that follow will indicate the approximate amount of wheatgrass that you will need prior to juicing. For optimal health, it's preferred to juice the wheatgrass separately and adding it to the mixer/blender with other nutrients such as the ones in this segment.

You can also purchase wheatgrass in other forms for convenience such as shown in some of the recipes also. For example, seven tablets or one rounded teaspoon of powder contains the nutrition of one serving of kale or spinach. You can receive the benefits without eating the veggies if you do not like them.

Other Things to Prepare:

- Add to weight loss shakes or smoothies (several included)
- Add to your favorite alcoholic beverage (1 is included)
- Add some of the wheatgrasses to macaroni or potato salad
- Add it to soups
- Add it to stews or any cooked meal

Breakfast

Banana Muffins

Ingredients:

- 1 t. of each:
    - Baking powder
    - Baking soda
- 1 ½ c. all-purpose flour
- ½ t. salt
- 1 egg
- 3 large mashed bananas
- ¾ c. white sugar
- 2 tbsp. Pines Wheatgrass
- 1/3 c. melted butter

How to Prepare:

1. Warm up the oven to 350°F.
2. Coat the muffin pans with some cooking spray or prepare with paper liners.
3. Sift/whisk the baking powder, flour, baking soda, and salt.
4. Combine the melted butter, egg, sugar, bananas, and wheatgrass in a large mixing bowl. Add to the prepared pans.
5. Bake the regular large muffins for 25–30 minutes or the mini muffins for 10–15 minutes. They should spring back when lightly pushed in the center.

Muesli With Berries—Wheatgrass & Kefir

Ingredients:

- 1 ½ c. kefir
- 4 tbsp. wheatgrass
- 1 1/3 c. fresh berries
- ½ t. cinnamon
- 1 t. honey

How to Prepare:

1. Toss the wheatgrass into a container and add the kefir. Sprinkle with the cinnamon and honey.
2. Rinse the berries and mix with the prepared wheatgrass and kefir.
3. Have a relaxing breakfast!

Porridge Additive

Ingredients:

- 1 t. of each:
    - Coconut oil
    - Wheatgrass powder
- ¾ c. coconut milk
- 3 tbsp. of each:
    - Almond flour/meal
    - Shredded/desiccated coconut
- 1 tbsp. of each:
    - Pumpkin seeds
    - Chia seeds
    - Flaxseed meal
- 1 pinch of salt
- ¼ t. vanilla extract

How to Prepare:

1. Combine the fixings in a small pan (low-med heat) and stir.
2. In a few minutes, the porridge will begin to thicken.
3. Add to a serving container when it is the way you like it.
4. Serve with the desired fruits or toppings.

Wheatgrass Oats

Ingredients:

- 2 tbsp. coconut flour
- 1 t. wheatgrass powder
- ½ c. cashew milk
- 1-2 egg whites
- ¼ t. vanilla extract
- 1/3 c. grated zucchini
- 2 droppers of vanilla crème
- 1 pinch of salt

How to Prepare:

1. Add all of the fixings in a small saucepan.
2. Stir while using the medium to low heat setting.
3. When ready, it will have an oatmeal consistency. Enjoy with your favorite toppings piping hot.

Lunch & Dinner

Carrot & Wheatgrass Salad

Ingredients:

- 1 large carrot
- 100 g wheatgrass, approximately 1 1/3 c.
- 400 g salad leaves, approximately 5 1/3 c.
- 1 t. of each:
    - Honey
    - Mustard
- 3 tbsp. sunflower oil

How to Prepare:

1. Shred the lettuce, leaving it in large chunks. Grate the carrot and mix both with the wheatgrass.
2. Give it all a sprinkle with the oil, honey, and mustard. If you like salt and pepper, add a bit of that as well.
3. Toss and enjoy!

Chicken Breasts Smothered in Wheatgrass

Ingredients:

- 4 pieces chicken breasts
- 1 onion
- 2 garlic cloves
- 1 egg
- 100 g. or approximately 1 1/3 c. of wheatgrass
- To Taste: Pepper & salt

How to Prepare:

1. Warm up the oven to 392°F.
2. Peel the onion and garlic. Grind in a blender along with the superfood. Blend in the egg.
3. Rub the breasts of chicken with pepper and salt and cover with the mixture.
4. Bake for about 20 minutes.
5. Serve and enjoy!

Green Salad

Ingredients:

- 1 large carrot
- 100 g./1 1/3 c. approximately ofwheatgrass
- 1 t. of each:
    - Honey
    - Mustard
- 400 g. salad leaves, approximately 5 1/3 c.

How to Prepare:

1. Tear the salad leaves into large chunks. Grate the carrot.
2. Mix the veggies with the wheatgrass. Sprinkle with the rest of the fixings and toss.
3. Feel free to add some pepper and salt to your liking.

Pesto Pizza

Ingredients:

- 1 c. fresh basil
- 1 pkg. pizza dough
- ¼ c. water
- 2 garlic cloves
- 2 tbsp. of each:
    - Olive oil
    - Pine nuts
- 2 t. wheatgrass powder
- 2 sliced tomatoes
- 8 oz. thinly sliced mozzarella

How to Prepare:

1. Program the oven setting to 450°F. Line a baking sheet with parchment paper.
2. Use a high-speed blender/food processor to combine the basil, wheatgrass powder, nuts, olive oil, and garlic. Pulse and add water a little at a time until it's like you like it.
3. Roll out the dough and arrange on the pizza sheet. Spread out the basil, cheese, and tomatoes.
4. Bake until the crust is browned and the cheese is melted (10-15 minutes).
5. Let it cool slightly before slicing.

Wheatgrass Tortillas With Ginger & Cumin

Ingredients:

- 1 small zucchini
- 1 t. cumin
- 100 g wheatgrass, approximately 1 1/3 c.
- ½ t. dried ginger powder
- To Taste: Salt

How to Prepare:

1. Thoroughly rinse the wheatgrass in water for 5 minutes. Grind it in a food processor. Grate the zucchini and blend with the superfood.
2. Fold in the rest of the fixings and salt as desired.
3. Toss on a few choice herbs before serving.

Dressings

Lime Cilantro Dressing

Ingredients:

- ½ avocado or ½ c. plain yogurt
- 1 c. loosely packed cilantro/coriander
- 2 tbsp. fresh lime juice
- 1 t. wheatgrass powder
- 1 clove of garlic
- ¼ c. olive oil
- 1 ½ t. apple cider vinegar
- 1/8 t. of each:
    - Cumin
    - Salt

How to Prepare:

1. Remove the stems from the cilantro and roughly chop. Juice the lime.
2. Combine all of the fixings in a food processor or blender.
3. Prepare until creamy smooth.
4. Make taste adjustments and enjoy.

Vinaigrette

Ingredients:

- 1 chopped garlic clove
- 3-inches wheatgrass, juiced
- 1 c. of each:
    - Extra-virgin olive oil
    - Rice vinegar/your favorite
- 1 t. cayenne pepper, if you like it hot
- ½ t. of each:
    - Salt
    - Black pepper/Crushed red pepper flakes

How to Prepare:

1. Combine all of the fixings in a container with a top or in a blender.
2. After preparing, store in a closed container in the fridge. It will be good for up to one week. Add your favorites and remember that the longer the flavors blend, the better the taste.

Desserts

Apples & Yogurt With Wheatgrass

Ingredients:

- Apple/another fruit of choice
- 1/3 c. wheatgrass
- 100 g. yogurt (1 1/3 c.)
- 1 t. honey

How to Prepare:

1. Steep the wheatgrass in a saucepan with enough water to cover the sprouted grains. Gently pour out the water.
2. Discard the apple peel and slice into small pieces.
3. Combine all of the fixings and enjoy!

Pineapple Wheatgrass Sorbet

Ingredients:

- 3 ½ c. ice
- 2 c. pineapple
- 1/3 c. agave
- 2 oz. fresh wheatgrass

How to Prepare:

1. Toss the wheatgrass and pineapple in a blender.
2. Puree until it is creamy.
3. Add the rest of the fixings and run until it's well blended.
4. You may need to place the sorbet in the freezer until it is firm.
5. *Note:* For a more citrusy drink, substitute a cup of lime juice in place of the pineapple.

Pumpkin Pie

Ingredients:

- 1 can (15 oz.) organic pumpkin puree
- 2 eggs
- 2 bananas
- ¼ c. coconut oil
- 1 c. coconut flour
- 1 tbsp. pumpkin pie spice
- ½ c. pecans
- 1-2 tbsp. green superfood powder—your choice
- 4 tbsp. maple syrup/agave/honey

How to Prepare:

1. Warm up the oven to 350°F.
2. Toss all of the fixings into a food processor.
3. Add the mixture into a 10-inch pie plate or a 6-x-8 glass dish.
4. Layer with a little coconut oil and bake for 20 minutes.
5. Let it cool and place in the fridge until ready to eat.

Pumpkin Spice Muffins

Ingredients:

- 2 tbsp. wheatgrass powder
- ½ c. pumpkin puree
- 4 eggs
- 4 bananas
- ¼ c. of each:
  - Almond butter
  - Maple syrup
- ½ c. coconut flour
- 4 tbsp. coconut oil
- 1 t. of each:
  - Pumpkin spice
  - Vanilla extract
  - Baking powder
- 1 pinch- salt

How to Prepare:

1. Preheat the oven to 350°F.
2. Use a food processor to blend all of the components of the muffin batter.
3. Pour the mixture into greased muffin tins (coconut oil).
4. Bake for 20 minutes.

Wheatgrass & Prunes Cookies

Ingredients:

- 2 tbsp. poppy seeds
- 1 ½ c. wheatgrass
- 100 g prunes (2/5 c.)

How to Prepare:

1. Combine the prunes and wheatgrass in a blender until the mixture is smooth.
2. Mix in the poppy seeds.
3. Shape the mixture into cookies and bake for 5 minutes (350°F). Rotate the cookies and cook for 5 more minutes.
4. *Note:* Watch closely so that it doesn't burn. Times can vary depending on the oven.

Chapter 7: Beverages & Smoothies With Wheatgrass

You can disguise the taste of wheatgrass in many ways, but a beverage, especially a smoothie, is the easiest way. You will also be receiving a pick-me-up whenever it is needed with one of these tasty drink choices:

Fruity Energy Shake

Ingredients:

- 1 banana
- 1 c. diced apple
- 1 c. crushed pineapple
- 2-inch round cut of wheatgrass

How to Prepare:

1. Add all of the components to your shaker. Mix well.
2. Take it with you if you are on the go. Enjoy anytime but store in the fridge.

Superfood Margarita

Ingredients:

- 8 oz. tequila
- 16 oz. unsweetened green tea
- 2 juiced limes
- 2 scoops wheatgrass powder
- 1 tbsp. agave nectar
- 1 sliced of each:
  - Jalapeno
  - Lime
  - Orange
  - Lemon

How to Prepare:

1. Use a large pitcher to mix the tea, tequila, lime juice, wheatgrass, and agave.
2. Add the sliced fixings, stir well, and serve in 4 chilled glasses.

Wheatgrass Latte

Ingredients:

- 1 c. almond/cashew/coconut milk
- 1 t. wheatgrass powder
- Optional: 2-3 drops Stevia/sweetener
- Also Needed: Aero-latte mixer

How to Prepare:

1. Combine all of the components. You can use a spoon to mix, but it is much easier with the Aero-latte.
2. *Note:* If you use a spoon, first, pour some milk into a glass and add 1 teaspoon of the wheatgrass. Make the paste and pour it in with the rest of the milk and combine well.
3. Enjoy as a soda replacement any time.

Wheatgrass-Nog

Ingredients:

- 1 banana
- 1 c. flax milk
- 1 t. of each:
    - Nutmeg
    - Cinnamon
- 2-3 dates/maple syrup
- 1 drop ginger oil
- 1 t.—1 tbsp. your choice wheatgrass powder

How to Prepare:

1. Mix all of the fixings in a blender.
2. Combine until creamy the way you like it.
3. Enjoy any time you want a taste change.

Wheatgrass Rejuvelac

Ingredients:

- 6 c. water
- ½ c. wheatgrass
- Also Needed: Cheesecloth

How to Prepare:

1. Prepare a 2-liter (67.628 oz.) bottle/jar or another liquid container with the wheatgrass in the bottom. Pour in the water.
2. Cover the jar/bottle with the cheesecloth and let it steep for three days.
3. *Note:* This is a non-alcoholic fermented beverage made from the sprouted grains. Your digestion is improved with the beneficial bacteria and healthy enzymes. It also contains as little as 20 calories for each cup.

Smoothies:

Apple & Banana Smoothie

Ingredients:

- 1 t. wheatgrass
- 3 over-ripened bananas
- Apple juice, 8 oz. or more (your choice)

How to Prepare:

1. Add the bananas in a hand blender or food processor to form a paste.
2. Add the rest of the fixings until it's the way you like it.

Banana, Green Mango, and Wheatgrass

Ingredients:

- ½ c. of each:
  - Pears
  - Unsweetened almond milk
- 1 small/med. frozen banana
- 1 c. spinach
- 1 t. wheatgrass powder
- 1 cilantro stem with leaves
- ¼ lime, juiced

How to Prepare:

1. Combine the ingredients in the blender jar.
2. Mix until smooth and serve in a chilled glass.

Blueberry Banana Smoothie

Ingredients:

- ½ banana
- 2 tbsp. presoaked chia seeds
- 1 c. of each:
    - Almond milk
    - Spinach
- ½ c. blueberries
- 1 tbsp. wheatgrass powder

How to Prepare:

1. Combine the fixings in the jar of a high-speed blender.
2. Mix until creamy smooth the way you like it.
3. Add a few ice cubes or pour over ice and enjoy!

Carrot Smoothie

Ingredients:

3 carrots
3-inch round wheatgrass
Water, for desired consistency
Ice cubes, to your liking

How to Prepare:

1. Simply add all of the fixings to a blender.
2. Add small amounts of water until it's how you like it.
3. Serve over ice or add ice to the blender.

Chocolate Banana Superfood Smoothie

Ingredients:

- 1 frozen, peeled, sliced banana
- 8 cubes of ice
- ½ c. spinach
- 1 can (13.5 oz.) full-fat coconut milk
- 1 tbsp. wheatgrass powder
- ½ t. vanilla extract
- 3 tbsp. of each:
    - Maple syrup
    - Cocoa powder

How to Prepare:

1. Prepare all of the fixings in a blender. Mix until it's creamy smooth.
2. Pour into a chilled glass and top it off with some fresh fruit or chia seeds for a healthy finish.
3. *Note:* Don't push this one aside because of the chocolate because it is full of elements that help fight against heart disease in relation to high blood pressure, blood clots, and cholesterol counts.

Green Smoothie

Ingredients:

- 2 celery stalks
- 2-3-inch round wheatgrass
- 1 c. spinach leaves
- 1/3 c. water
- ½ c. parsley

How to Prepare:

1. Blend all of the ingredients and enjoy.
2. You can add ice cubes to the smoothies or blend them during preparation.

Green–Blueberry Smoothie

Ingredients:

- 1 banana
- 1 c. of each:
- Flaxseed milk
- Blueberries
- 1 tbsp. of each:
    - Pines wheatgrass powder
    - Hempseed oil

How to Prepare:

1. Combine the components in a blender.
2. Serve over ice cubes and relax.

Green Tea Party Smoothie

Ingredients:

- 12 oz. hot water
- 1 bag green tea
- 4 large pieces of kale
- 1 c. frozen berries
- 1 banana, frozen & peeled
- 2 tbsp. almonds
- ¼ c. regular/gluten-free rolled oats
- 1 tbsp. wheatgrass powder
- Optional: 2 Medjool dates
- 1 c. ice

How to Prepare:

1. Prepare the green tea and cool. Combine with the rest of the fixings.
2. Blend until smooth and enjoy any time.

Kiwi Detox Smoothies for 4

Ingredients:

- 2 limes, juiced
- 4 kiwi fruits
- 2 tbsp. mint leaves
- 3 tbsp. snipped wheatgrass
- 1 tbsp. apple juice
- ½ c. ice cubes
- 1 handful leafy green such as spinach

How to Prepare:

1. Peel and chop the kiwi and add to a blender along with the lime juice and wheatgrass.
2. Chop the mint and add. Toss in the ice and blend. Add enough juice to make it the desired consistency you crave.
3. Enjoy in 4 frosty glasses.

Mint Choco-Chip Smoothie

Ingredients:

- 1 frozen banana
- 1 c. spinach
- 1 ½ c. almond/cashew/coconut milk
- ½ avocado
- 2 handfuls mint
- 1 t. wheatgrass powder
- 1 tbsp. cacao nibs
- Optional for Serving: Coconut whipped cream

How to Prepare:

1. Blend all of the fixings in a blender (omit the nibs for now).
2. Once mixed, add the nibs and pulse a time or two.
3. Transfer to a chilled glass with the whipped cream and a sprinkle of the cacao nibs.
4. Enjoy anytime you want to avoid a sugary treat.

Pineapple Smoothie

Ingredients:

- 1 frozen banana
- 1 c. of each:
    - Frozen pineapple
    - Juice/milk
- ½-1 tbsp. Pines Wheatgrass, to your liking

How to Prepare

1. Combine all of the ingredients in a blender.
2. Mix well until it is the texture desired.
3. Serve over ice in a chilled glass.

Simply Tangy Wheatgrass Smoothie

Ingredients:

- 2 juiced oranges
- 1 juiced lime
- 1 banana
- 3-inch round wheatgrass
- 2 c. crushed ice

How to Prepare:

1. Blend the juices and toss the ice into a blender.
2. Serve in chilled glasses.
3. Enjoy as a midafternoon treat.

Vanilla Soy Wheatgrass Smoothie

Ingredients:

- ¼ banana
- ½ c. vanilla soy milk
- ¼ c. frozen berries of your choice
- 1 t. of each:
    - Wheatgrass powder
    - Honey
- 1 shake of cinnamon

How to Prepare:

1. Toss all of the fixings in a blender.
2. Mix until smooth and serve.

Vegan Smoothie With Peanut Butter

Ingredients:

- 1 large handful spinach
- 1 very ripe banana
- ½ c. almond milk
- 1 heaping tbsp. peanut butter
- To your Liking:
    - Ginger
    - Cinnamon
    - Chia seeds
- 1 ¼ t. Pines Wheatgrass Powder

How to Prepare:

1. Add all of the fixings to the blender.
2. Combine until well blended and enjoy.

Veggie Smoothie

Ingredients:

- ½ of a beetroot
- 2 carrots
- 3 large celery stalks
- 4 inches wheatgrass
- ½ c. of each:
    - Fresh parsley
    - Alfalfa sprouts/your choice of sprouts
- 2 c. fresh spinach leaves

How to Prepare:

1. Combine all of the fixings in a blender.
2. Serve knowing you are receiving a healthy smoothie.

You can adapt this recipe with your favorite veggies. The choices are unlimited.

Conclusion

Thanks for viewing your copy of *Wheatgrass: The Guidebook for Enjoying a World of Health Benefits of a Superfood.* Let's hope it was informative and provided you with all of the tools you need to achieve your goals no matter what they may be. You know the superfood will provide you with so many benefits—how can you go wrong? The answer is: you can't go wrong.

If your life is busy shuffling school, children, or work, the wheatgrass juice may be just what you need. Give it a try using some of these great recipes. You will probably adjust to the taste when mixed with other foods. The next step is to recall the essential foods you would like to incorporate using wheatgrass—the Superfood.

Finally, if you found this book useful in any way, a review on Amazon is always appreciated!

Index of Recipes

Chapter 6: Quality Foods Using Wheatgrass

Breakfast:

1. Banana Muffins
2. Muesli with Berries—Wheatgrass & Kefir
3. Porridge Additive
4. Wheatgrass Oats

Lunch & Dinner

1. Carrot & Wheatgrass Salad
2. Chicken Breasts Smothered in Wheatgrass
3. Green Salad
4. Pesto Pizza
5. Wheatgrass Tortillas With Ginger & Cumin

Dressings

1. Lime Cilantro Dressing
2. Vinaigrette

Desserts

1. Apples & Yogurt With Wheatgrass
2. Pineapple Wheatgrass Sorbet
3. Pumpkin Pie
4. Pumpkin Spice Muffins
5. Wheatgrass & Prunes Cookies

Chapter 7: Beverages & Smoothies With Wheatgrass

1. Fruity Energy Shake
2. Superfood Margarita
3. Wheatgrass Latte
4. Wheatgrass-Nog
5. Wheatgrass Rejuvelac

Smoothies:

1. Apple & Banana Smoothie
2. Banana—Green Mango & Wheatgrass Smoothie
3. Blueberry Banana Smoothie
4. Carrot Smoothie